“WHEN NOTHING WORKS:

A 3-DAY FAST FOR DELIVERANCE, DIRECTION, AND DIVINE REALIGNMENT”

REV. DR. MARIE BREVIL

This book is a work of sacred intention. It is designed for personal transformation, reflection, and healing.

The prayers, affirmations, rituals, and writings contained herein are not intended to replace professional medical, mental health, or spiritual counsel.

Unless otherwise stated, all scripture references, rituals, affirmations, and prayers are original works authored by Dr. Brevil. Any resemblance to other works is purely coincidental or drawn from universal spiritual wisdom shared across cultures.

Published by My Littl' Workshop
NY & PA, USA

First Edition: 2025

Cover Design: Marie Brevil
Interior Layout: Marie Brevil

Printed in the USA

For permissions, collaborations, or speaking inquiries, contact:

Rev. Dr. Marie Brevil
My Littl' Workshop

Name:

Gift from:

Year:

Misc.:

INTRODUCTION

Introduction: When Nothing Works – the Meaning of This Book

There comes a moment in life when words fall short, when plans crumble, when the very ground beneath you feels unstable. You've cried, prayed, strategized, worked hard, trusted, and still... nothing has changed. The job is gone. The relationship broke. The investment failed. The betrayals cut deep. And what once gave you purpose or peace now feels like a distant memory.

This book is for that moment.

It is for when you're feeling sad, unaccomplished, and uncertain.

For when your chest is heavy with silence.

For when you've done all you could do and yet, life still refuses to open.

INTRODUCTION

It is for the nights that blur into mornings without answers.

For the heartbreak that feels like it will never end.

For the confusion that paralyzes the next step.

For the hope that feels foolish and the faith that feels fragile.

INTRODUCTION

This book is a spiritual tool. A sacred guide. A fast for deliverance, for renewal, and for realignment.
It is not about blaming others or demanding pity.
It is not about temporary motivation or surface-level healing.
It is for those ready to rise.
This is for when you finally say:

"Enough is enough."

When you become willing to try something new – not to impress anyone, not to get attention, but to consecrate yourself back to your own soul.

This book holds a 3-day fast – a journey of spiritual warfare and deliverance – for when everything else has failed. It's a fast to address spiritual attacks, break inner and outer bondages, and restore your divine alignment.

You will fast. You will pray.
You will affirm truth into your bones.
You will ask yourself questions no one else can ask for you.

YOU WILL...

You will cry and release, invoke and declare, forgive and rise.

And then – you will know.

Because this book isn't just for when nothing works.

It's for when you're ready to work with God and finally heal, face your truth, and walk differently.

So come open. Come broken. Come exhausted if that's where you are.

But come willing. Come ready. Come consecrated to your change.

It begins here.

And it begins with you.

WHEN NOTHING WORKS – TRY THIS

When Nothing Works – Try This
This is not just a book.
This is a turning point.

This fast is for the big change – the one you've been praying for, dreaming of, waiting on. The one that feels long overdue.
The one that shakes the ground beneath your feet not to destroy you, but to finally rebuild you.

You've tried.
You've cried.

You've shown up again and again.
But somehow – life just isn't moving.
And now, you're here.
Not for another motivational fix.
Not for another trend.

But because your soul is whispering:
"Do something different...for you."

INTRODUCTION

This is a spiritually grounded 3-day fast for elevation, deliverance, and breakthrough – a sacred space for when you feel spiritually stuck, physically drained, mentally foggy, emotionally wounded, or under attack in ways no one else seems to understand.

It's for the moment you reach your wit's end.
When nothing seems to be working.
When the people you trusted turn away.
When betrayal, failure, stagnation, heartbreak, and spiritual confusion seem to meet you at every corner.
And now... you're ready.

You're not just hoping for change anymore.
You're creating space for it.
You're ready for a spiritual shift that's deeper, purer, and truer than anything you've experienced before.

THIS BOOK IS FOR YOU IF:

This book is for you if:

- You feel spiritually under attack.
- You've been betrayed, backstabbed, or broken.
- You feel like you've given so much and received so little.
- You want clarity – not chaos.
- You need a break from the noise and need something real.
- You're ready for results, not just routines.

Why Fasting?

Because fasting clears the fog – spiritually and physically.

It is not just some spiritual ritual or religious performance. It's a tool. A weapon. A divine reset.

Fasting clears your mind, sharpens your spirit, and re-centers your soul. It cuts through the noise. It lifts the frequency. It breaks bondages and ignites truth. It teaches you to hear again – not from the world, but from within.

CONT'D

And it's common sense too:

A lighter body brings a lighter mind.

A clearer head leads to wiser decisions.

A rested spirit sees through illusions and stands in truth.

BUT LET'S BE HONEST

But let's be honest – fasting is not for the lazy.

It is for those who are serious.

For those ready to take responsibility, stop blaming, and begin deep inner work.

To truly approach this fast, you must:

- Let go of excuses.
- Stop blaming others and start reflecting inward.
- Be honest about your regrets, patterns, and choices.
- Surrender fully – no shortcuts, no sidesteps.
- Commit to being spiritually present and grounded every step of the way.

STRUCTURING YOUR FAST

Everyone's fast will look different.

Some will do it with water only, others with juices, broth, shakes, or fruits and vegetables. You choose what works for your body and soul – this is about spiritual focus and integrity, not copying someone else's path.

The most important thing is that you:

- Commit to your method.
- Honor your intention.
- Don't shift your plan because of others' opinions.
- Remember why you started – especially when it gets uncomfortable.

Don't let the gaslighting, the outside noise, or the fear of judgment intimidate you. This is your fast. Your fight. Your spiritual reclamation.

STRUCTURING YOUR FAST

So decide.
Then do it.

You're not here by accident.
You're not broken beyond repair.

You're just overdue for a shift.

Let this fast be your sacred reset.

Let this book walk you home.

TRY THIS...

When Nothing Works – Try This

There comes a time in life when everything feels like it's falling apart.

Your business fails.
The job is gone.
Your lover lied.
Your home is lost.
The investment didn't go through.

You gave your all,
and somehow it still wasn't enough.

You tried different paths.
You prayed.
You listened.
You waited.

You showed up,
hoping it would turn around.
But still – nothing changed.
And now, you've arrived
at a breaking point.

WHEN NOTHING WORKS – TRY THIS

There comes a time in life when everything feels like it's falling apart.

Your business fails.
The job is gone.
Your lover lied.
Your home is lost.
The investment didn't go through.

You gave your all,
and somehow it still wasn't enough.

You tried different paths.
You prayed or invoked.
You listened.
You waited.

You showed up,
hoping it would turn around.
But still – nothing changed.
And now, you've arrived
at a breaking point.

THIS BOOK IS FOR...

This book is for that moment.

When you feel sad, unaccomplished, overwhelmed.

When you feel like you've done all you can, and yet nothing seems to work.

When the emptiness speaks louder than your plans.

When you are ready to say – "Enough is enough."

"ENOUGH IS ENOUGH."

When you are ready to say – "Enough is enough."

This is not a casual read.

This is a sacred manual for transformation.

This is a 3-day spiritually grounded fast for those who are finally ready for breakthrough – real breakthrough.

The kind that shifts timelines.

The kind that breaks generational bondage.

The kind that elevates your spirit and changes the direction of your life.

WHAT THIS FAST IS FOR

This fast is for those who want real change.

Not temporary motivation.
Not surface-level healing.

But the deep, divine change that uproots the old and plants something sacred in its place.

This is for those who feel like they've done the work but aren't seeing the return.

For those who feel spiritually stuck or attacked.

For the weary, the wounded, the betrayed.

For those whose hearts are heavy, whose spirits are tired, and whose minds feel clouded.

WHAT THIS FAST IS FOR

This fast is for you if you're ready to:

- Let go of all that no longer serves you
- Cut cords with the past and toxic patterns
- Reclaim your voice, your power, your clarity
- Elevate into a new level of spiritual awareness
- Be consistent in your peace, your choices, your boundaries
- Stop begging and start believing

This fast is a decision to start anew – fully, unapologetically, and spiritually grounded.

WHY FASTING?

Why Fasting?

Because when you fast – you clear the fog.

You create space.

You cut through the mental clutter, the spiritual noise, the emotional overload.

Fasting allows your body to reset and your spirit to rise.

It is not just about food – it's about focus.

When your body is light, your spirit is sharp.

When your stomach is quiet, your soul can finally speak.

This is not superstition.
This is alignment.

WHY FASTING?

Fasting clears the mind.
Fasting sharpens the spirit.
Fasting detoxes the soul.

Fasting helps you see what was already inside of you – now without distraction.

It doesn't matter if you're fasting for spiritual warfare, emotional clarity, or energetic reset – the result is the same:

Clarity.

Power.

Peace.

WHY FASTING?

How to Truly Approach This Fast

To receive the fullness of this journey, you must be willing to do the real work. This isn't about starving yourself.
It's about consecration.
It's about devotion. It's about letting go of blame and stepping fully into responsibility.

You must decide:

- To stop avoiding what needs to be faced
- To stop blaming others for your delays
- To be honest about your own patterns
- To surrender to the process without shortcuts
- To show up for yourself as if your life depends on it — because it does

Let this fast be your reset. Let it be sacred. Let it be intentional. Let it be real.

WHY FASTING?

Types of Fast – Choose Your Way

This fast can be tailored to your body's needs and your spirit's wisdom. You don't need to copy anyone's method. You're invited to tune into yourself and structure your fast according to what aligns.

Here are some options:

- Water fast (pure water only)
- Juice fast (fruit or vegetable juices only)
- Raw fruit and vegetable fast
- Liquid fast (includes smoothies, shakes, herbal teas, broths, or bouillons)
- Bone broth or soup-based fast

There is no one-size-fits-all.
What matters most is intentionality.
Set your standard. Choose your path.
And then – commit.

WHY FASTING?

Your Fast. Your Fight. Your Healing.

Do not let others talk you out of your healing.

Do not be swayed by opinions, judgments, or fear.

Do not dim your light for people who didn't show up for your pain.

You do you.
This is your sacred reset.
Your spiritual realignment.
Your internal uprising.
Remember why you began this fast in the first place.
Don't forget your reason. Don't abandon your commitment.
Not for fear. Not for guilt. Not for anyone.
When you fast – fast for your healing.

Fast for your clarity.
Fast for your future.

LET THIS BE THE MOMENT

Let This Be the Moment
Let this be the day you rise.

Let this be the fast that shifts everything.

Let this be the sacred pause that changes the rest of your journey.

You don't just believe anymore – now you know.

And that knowing changes everything.

INTRODUCTION

There are moments in life when you feel like you've tried everything and nothing works. You've put in effort, time, and faith, but the outcomes remain the same—disappointing, draining, and unclear. That sense of stagnation can lead to frustration, sadness, and even hopelessness. You begin to question whether change is even possible, and you wonder what else can be done.

This book was written for that exact moment.

It is for when you're feeling unaccomplished, unsure, and stuck. It's for when you've tried different paths, but none have brought the healing or transformation you hoped for. It's for when your spirit is heavy, your heart is tired, and you are finally ready to say, "Enough is enough."

INTRODUCTION

This is not about religion or ritual for the sake of tradition. This is about spiritual grounding. It's about reconnecting with yourself and realigning your mind, body, and spirit. This book offers a three-day fasting journey—not just for discipline, but for elevation. A sacred reset, initiated by you, for you.

WHAT THIS FAST IS FOR

What This Fast Is For

This fast is designed for those seeking real, lasting change. It's for individuals who have tried many things but still feel stuck, unseen, unheard, or unfulfilled. You may feel spiritually blocked, emotionally overwhelmed, or physically exhausted. Maybe you've invested time and energy in your growth, but the results don't match your efforts. If you feel like nothing you've done has led to the breakthrough you're looking for, this may be the shift you've been waiting on.

This fast is especially helpful for those navigating spiritual attacks, emotional trauma, betrayal, burnout, or internal conflict.

WHAT THIS FAST IS FOR

It’s also appropriate for those who feel like they’re reaching a point of collapse —mentally, spiritually, or physically— and are now ready to reclaim their power.

If you're looking for clarity, renewal, and a deeper connection with yourself and your Creator, this fast is the right place to start. It is not about complicating your life with rigid rules.

On the contrary, it’s about stripping things down to what matters and what works. This fast is for those seeking simplicity with power, and depth without confusion.

WHY FASTING?

Why Fasting?

Fasting is a tool that's been used for centuries to clear the mind, purify the body, and connect deeply with the spirit. It's not about deprivation—it's about realignment. It helps you cut through noise, both internally and externally. It offers you the space and clarity to reset your thoughts, regulate your emotions, and recenter your intentions.

Fasting allows your body to rest from constant digestion, which in turn allows your mind to focus and your spirit to heighten. This is not just about health, although health benefits are a strong bonus. Fasting can elevate your mental clarity, emotional resilience, and spiritual awareness.

This is not about magic or superstition —it's about biology, rhythm, and energetic alignment.

WHY FASTING?

A clear body supports a clear mind. A clear mind allows you to think wisely, make sound decisions, and hear your inner guidance. Fasting is a tool for healing and for elevation, both practically and spiritually.

HOW TO APPROACH THIS FAST

How to Approach This Fast

If you're serious about using this fast as a tool for transformation, then it's important to approach it with intention and discipline. This isn't about punishing your body or rushing the process. It's about making a decision to shift. That requires accountability, not blame; responsibility, not excuses.

Start by being honest with yourself. This fast will likely bring up things you've been avoiding. That's part of the healing process. You will need to release old patterns, surrender your resistance, and stay committed to your intention. You must be willing to face discomfort and grow from it.

HOW TO APPROACH THIS FAST

There are no shortcuts here. If you approach this process passively, it won't yield the results you want. You are the one responsible for your healing. This fast is an act of devotion—to yourself and your future. Treat it as such.

HOW TO APPROACH THIS FAST

Structuring Your Fast

This is not a one-size-fits-all method. People come into fasting with different needs, health conditions, and spiritual experiences. That's why this process should be adapted to fit what's best for you.

Some people will fast with water only. Others may choose juice, herbal teas, vegetable broth, or nutrient-dense smoothies. Others might use only raw fruits and vegetables. You may combine elements to suit your health and spiritual goals.

The key is to make a clear decision before you begin. Set your boundaries.

HOW TO APPROACH THIS FAST

Decide what you are abstaining from and why. Be consistent. Stay grounded in your reason for doing this fast in the first place.

Do not let other people's opinions confuse your path. You do not need to explain your journey to anyone. Don't alter your fast to make others more comfortable. This is your healing, your process, and your responsibility.

BEFORE YOU BEGIN

Final Thoughts Before You Begin

You are here because you're ready for something more. Something deeper. Something real. This fast is your opportunity to reset from the inside out.

Be honest about what you need. Be clear about what you're releasing. Be intentional about what you're calling in.

Don't let fear, fatigue, or the opinions of others pull you away from what you know you need. You are allowed to prioritize yourself. You are allowed to heal. You are allowed to grow. And you are allowed to do it in a way that works for you.

This journey will require focus, courage, and consistency. But if you commit, it will change your life.
Now, let's begin.

THE ARC OF INNER WORK:

Flow of the 3 Days (The Arc of Inner Work):

1. Day 1: You meet your past face-to-face – reflect, admit, take ownership.
2. Day 2: You let go of what no longer serves – forgive, release, and declare your new self.
3. Day 3: You step forward with joy – give thanks, rebuild trust, and begin again.

During this journey, some will call it prayer, others will call it invocation or even treatment. Don't be distracted, stay focused on the tasks and your journey.

NOTES

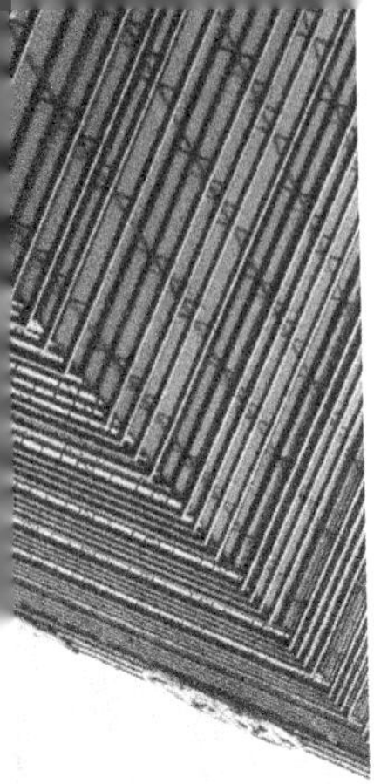

DAY 1:

Day 1: "Pulling the Past Forward"

Theme: Reflection, Responsibility, and Acknowledgment

Definition:

This day is about looking at your past honestly—not to get stuck there, but to understand its impact and bring the lessons to the surface.

It's about reflecting on your story, taking responsibility for what you can change, and acknowledging the truths you've avoided, denied, or dimmed.

Why It Matters:

You cannot heal what you won't look at. If you don't pull the past forward consciously, it will keep pulling you backward subconsciously.

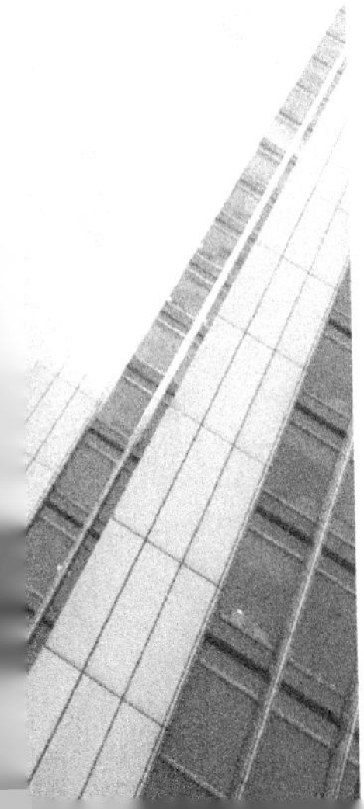

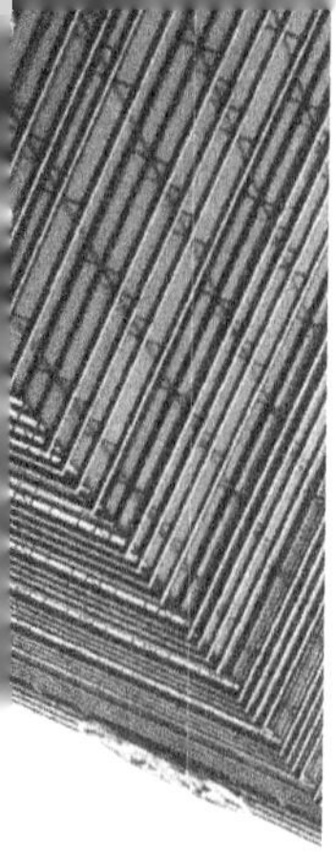

DAY 1:

Example:

You were abandoned emotionally as a child. For years, you overextended yourself in relationships trying to earn love.

Day 1 is where you acknowledge this pattern without shame. You say: "Yes, this is what happened. Yes, it shaped me. But now I choose to learn from it instead of being ruled by it."

This is not about blame. This is about owning your response moving forward.
✧ "When you look back with eyes of power instead of pain, you begin the process of transformation."

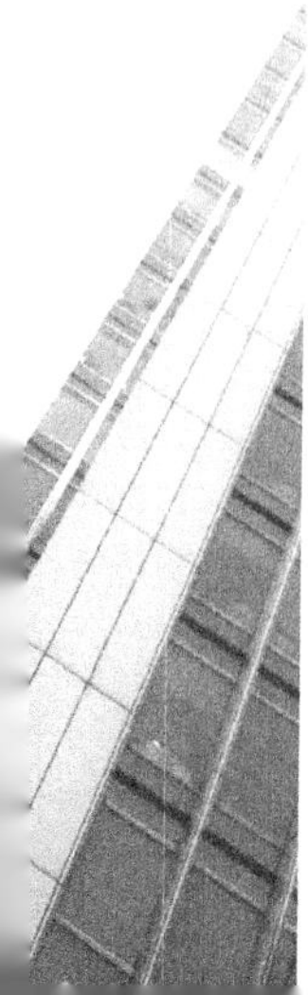

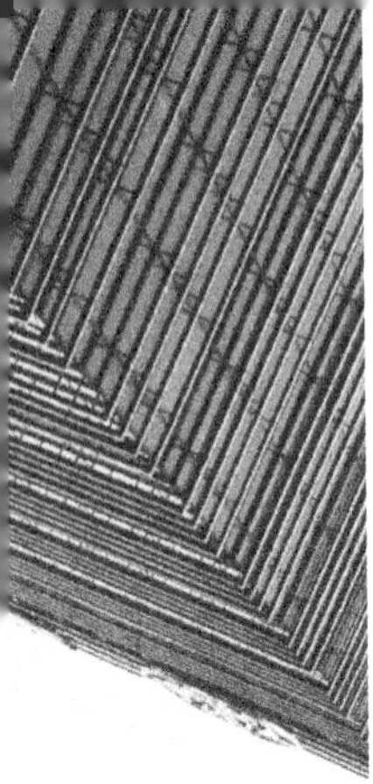

DAY 1:

Pulling the Past Forward

Theme: Reflection, Responsibility, and Acknowledgment

Focus: What needs to be let go of? What cycles are you repeating? Why is this happening?

There can be no true elevation without confrontation. Day 1 invites you to take an honest look at what has followed you into this moment—consciously or unconsciously.

This is the day to bring forward the patterns, behaviors, and beliefs that have held you back, so they can finally be addressed, acknowledged, and released.

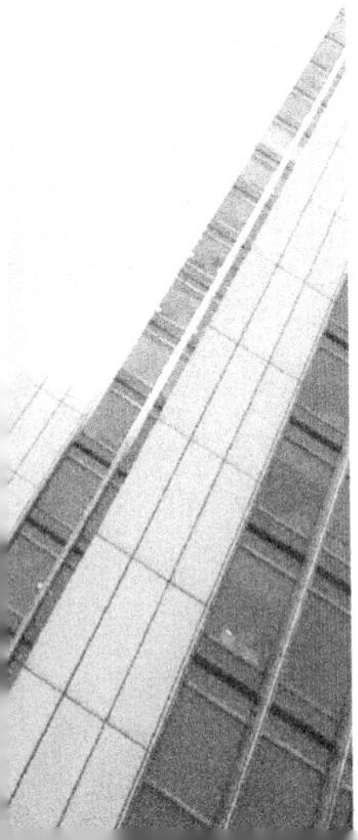

You cannot heal what you do not face. You cannot shift what you are not willing to confront.

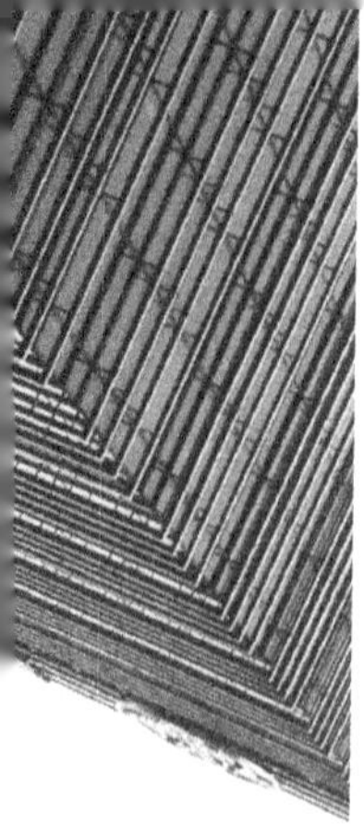

DAY 1:

The cycles that keep repeating in your life are not coincidences—they are unhealed echoes of your past, asking to be understood and transmuted.

This day asks you to stand still, look inward, and be brave enough to sit with the weight of your truth—not to be punished by it, but to be freed through it. You are here because you're ready to stop running and start reclaiming.

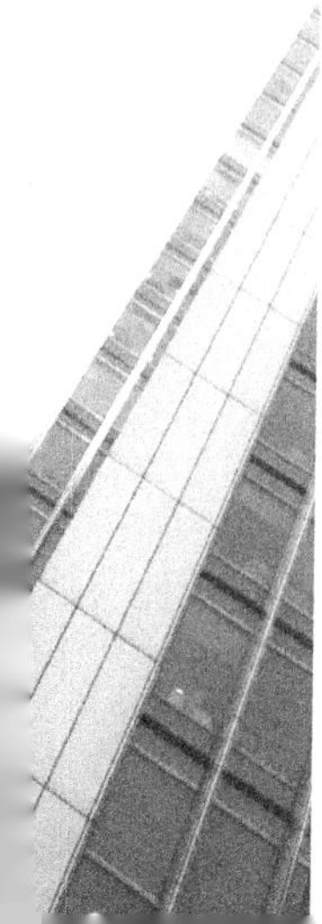

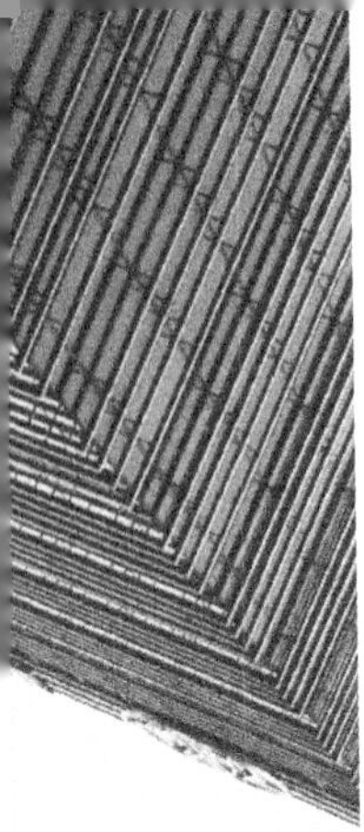

DAY 1:

Prayer/Invocation for Clarity and Self-Revelation

Dear Divine Source,
I come before you in this sacred moment asking for the clarity I cannot give myself. Remove the fog that clouds my understanding. Illuminate the truth I need to see, even if I've been too afraid to look at it.

Grant me the courage to see beyond distractions, beyond comfort, and into the essence of who I've become. Show me what I've normalized that is no longer serving me. Help me recognize the difference between what is familiar and what is healthy.

Call in the forces that walk in light, that honor healing, that support my higher journey. May they guide my steps with wisdom and anchor me in a sense of purpose far deeper than appearances.

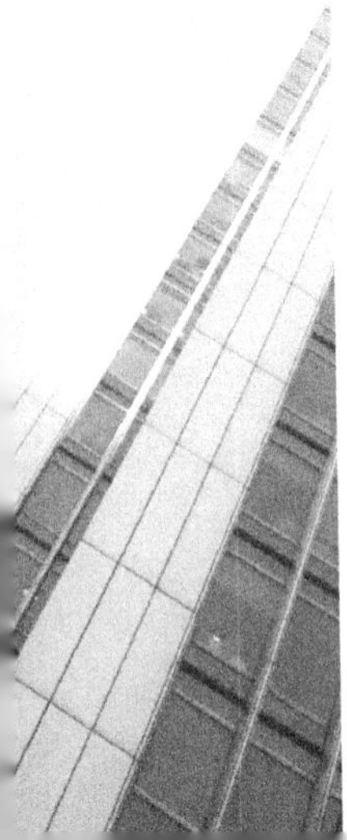

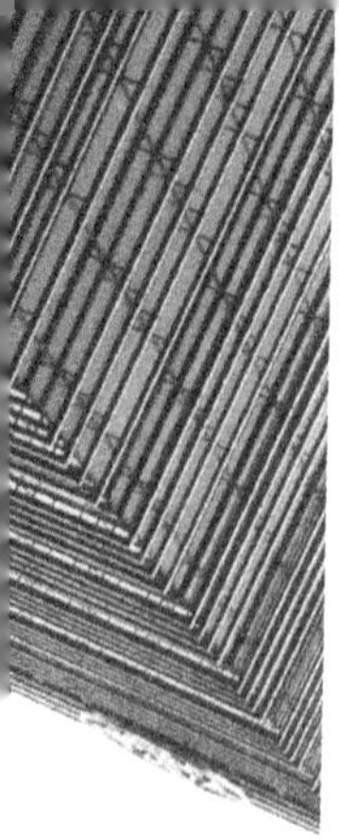

DAY 1:

This is a sacred path I walk—not just for healing, but for transformation. Help me walk it with reverence. Let me rise beyond the ordinary, and into the truth I was born to carry.

Amen.

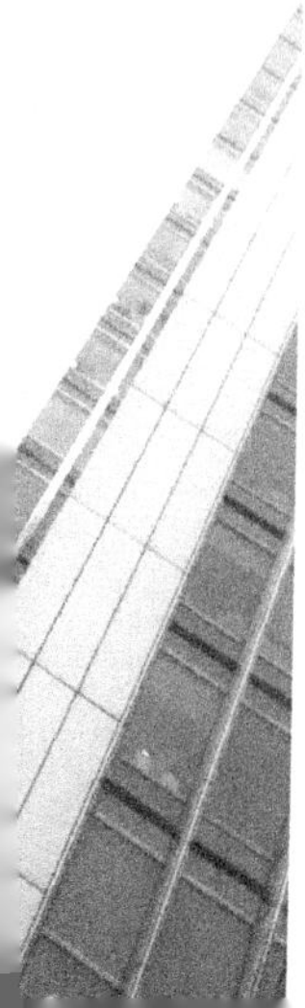

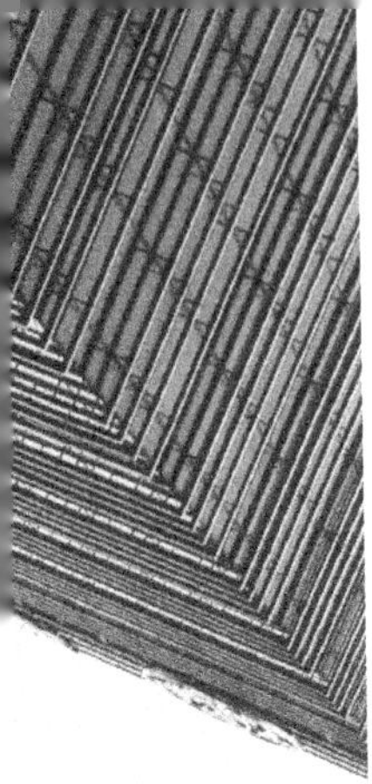

DAY 1:

Prayer for Strength to Face the Truth

Holy One,

You know how long I've hidden from certain truths. You know how often I've chosen denial over clarity, comfort over confrontation, silence over healing. But I no longer want to run from what needs to be faced.

Grant me strength—not just physical, but emotional and spiritual—to sit with what's been buried. Help me face the truths that feel too raw to touch. Remind me that truth, even when painful, is not punishment. It is the pathway to peace.

Let your truth rise in me like the sun—gentle, consistent, undeniable. Strip away illusions.

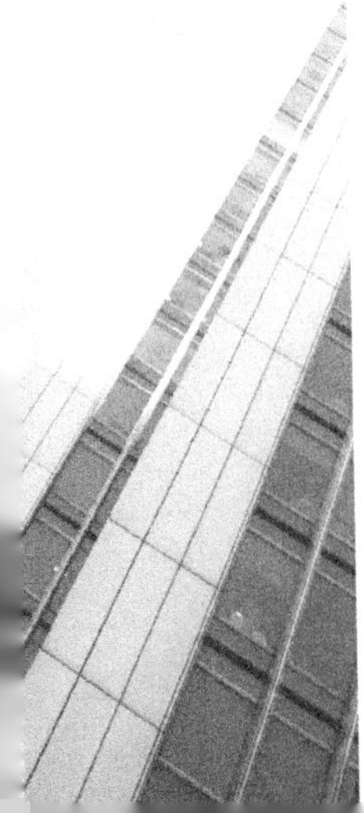

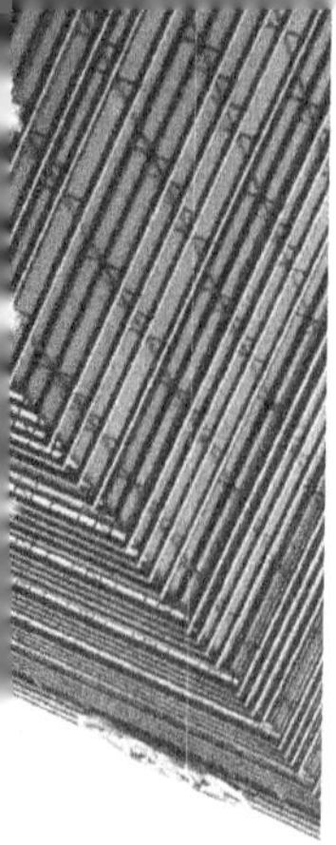

DAY 1:

Bring forward what is real, what is pure, and what must be seen in order for me to be free.

May I meet my truth with grace, not shame. With reverence, not regret. With love, not fear.

Amen.

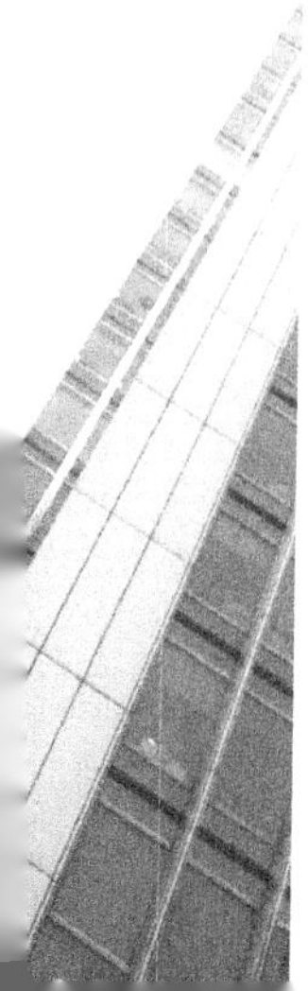

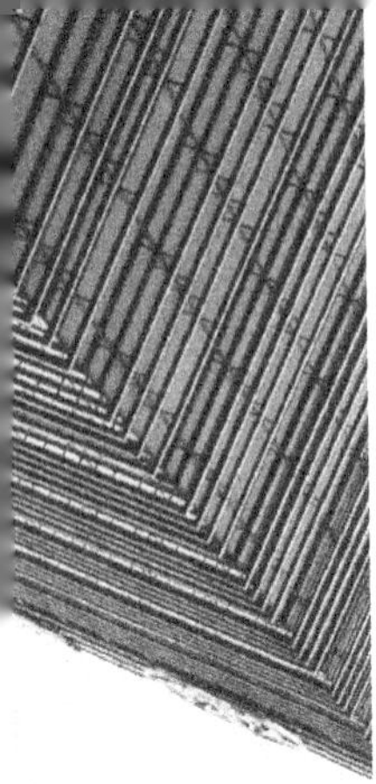

DAY 1:

Prayer to Break the Spirit of Self-Sabotage

Spirit of Life,

I confess: I have gotten in my own way. I have spoken against myself, doubted my worth, and denied my greatness. I have delayed my healing. I have looked outward for someone to blame, when the work I needed to do was within.

Today, I choose something different.

I renounce every habit, mindset, and belief that causes me to sabotage my progress. I break every agreement I've made—spoken or unspoken—that says I am unworthy of success, peace, or joy.

Reveal to me the roots of my self-sabotage. Help me uproot every pattern I've normalized. Bring healing to the wounds that created them.

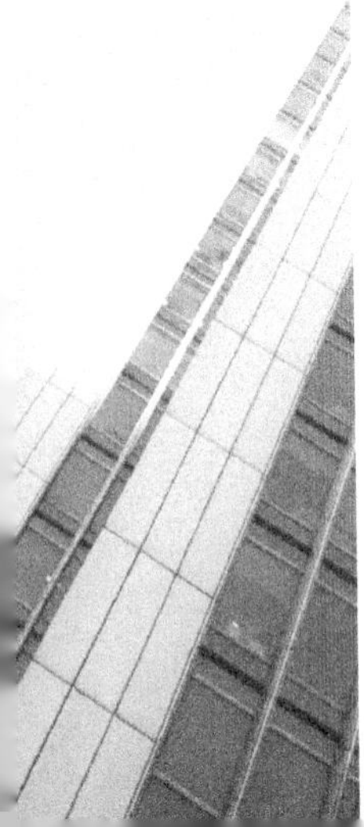

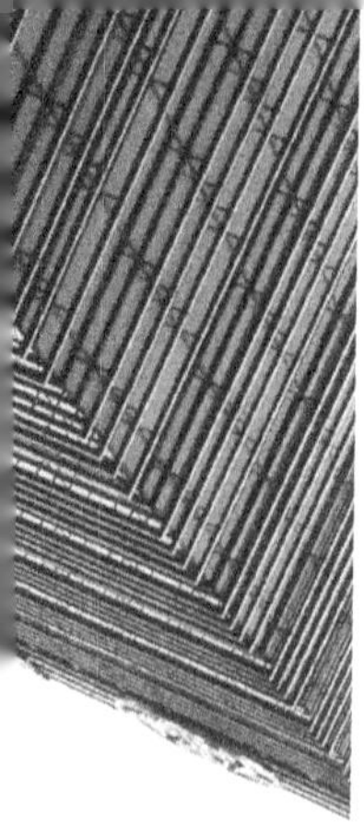

DAY 1:

I accept responsibility for my life from this point forward. I give myself permission to be powerful, whole, and ready.

I will no longer be my own obstacle.

Amen.

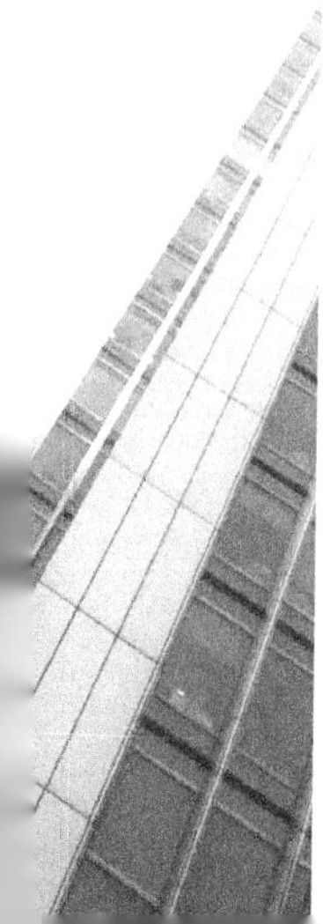

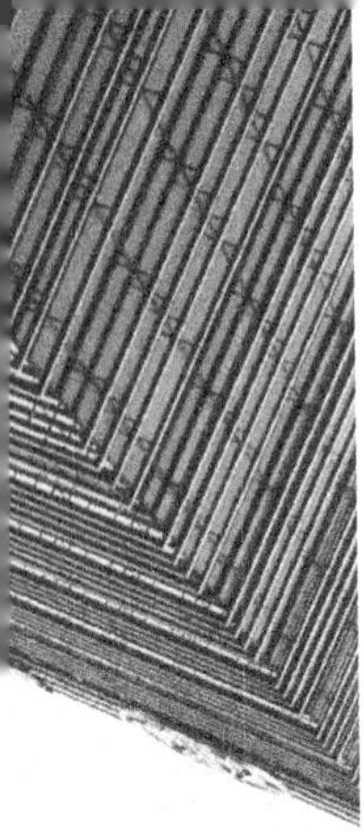

DAY 1:

33 Affirmations for Day 1

1. I am not my past.
2. I am allowed to change.
3. Every mistake teaches me something sacred.
4. I face my truth with love.
5. I forgive myself for what I did not know.
6. My healing matters.
7. I am ready to move forward.
8. I release the guilt that no longer serves me.
9. I accept myself fully.
10. I choose growth over stagnation.
11. I trust myself to do the work.
12. My past prepared me, it did not define me.
13. I let go of the blame.
14. I take full ownership of my life.
15. I deserve peace.
16. I see the patterns and I choose to change them.

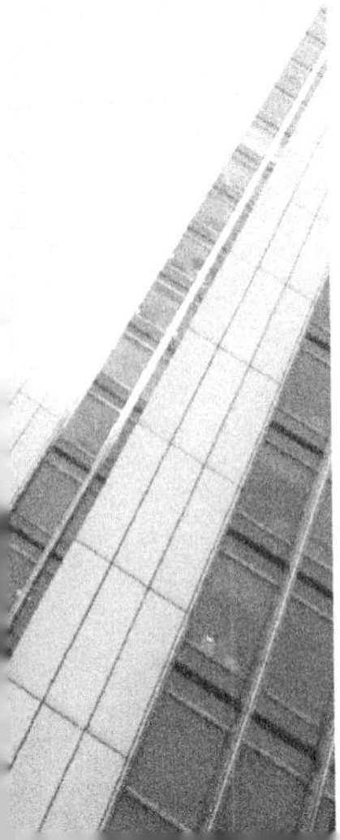

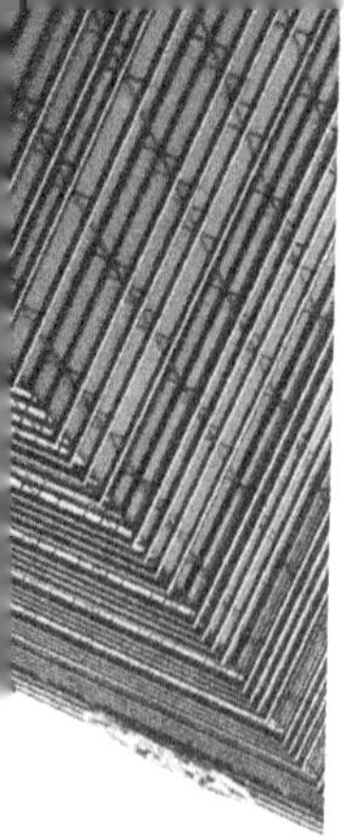

DAY 1:

17. I welcome new beginnings.
18. I can heal from anything.
19. I treat myself with compassion.
20. I honor the journey that brought me here.
21. I break every cycle that keeps me small.
22. My mind is clear and open.
23. I am rooted in truth.
24. I trust divine timing.
25. I listen to my intuition.
26. I have the power to change my story.
27. I am enough.
28. I accept all parts of my journey.
29. I no longer hide from myself.
30. I speak life into my soul.
31. I release the past with grace.
32. I align myself with healing.
33. I walk forward in love and power.

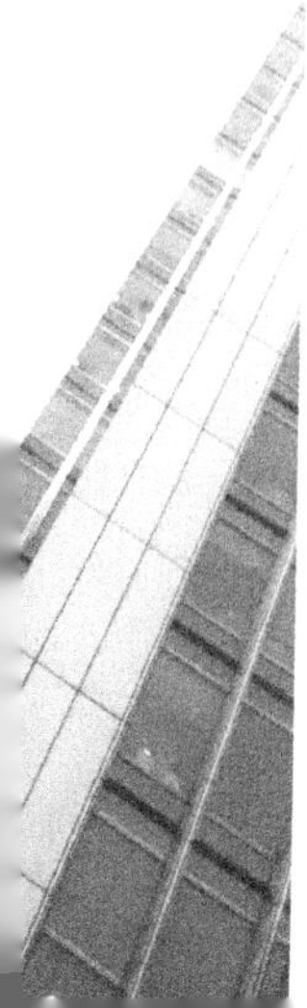

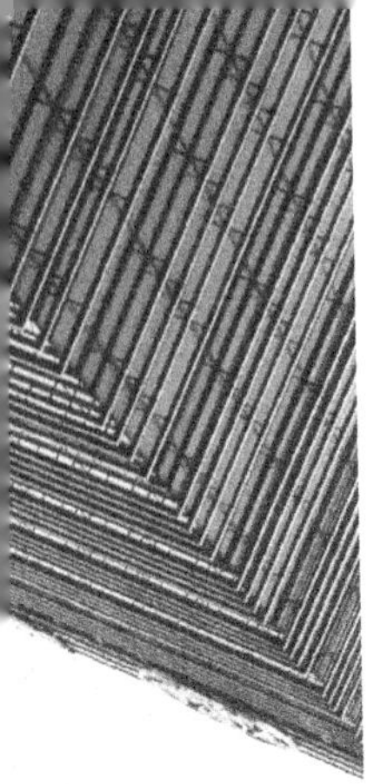

DAY 1:

33 Deep Questions for Reflection and Journaling

1. What patterns have I seen repeat in my life?
2. What emotions do I often suppress or ignore?
3. What do I regret, and how can I honor that pain without living in it?
4. Who have I blamed for my suffering, and what does that reveal about my inner wounds?
5. What does forgiveness mean to me?
6. What would I do differently if I believed I was truly worthy?
7. What was the hardest truth I've ever had to face about myself?
8. What am I still holding onto that no longer serves me?
9. When did I first begin to doubt my voice?
10. What experiences shaped my self-worth?

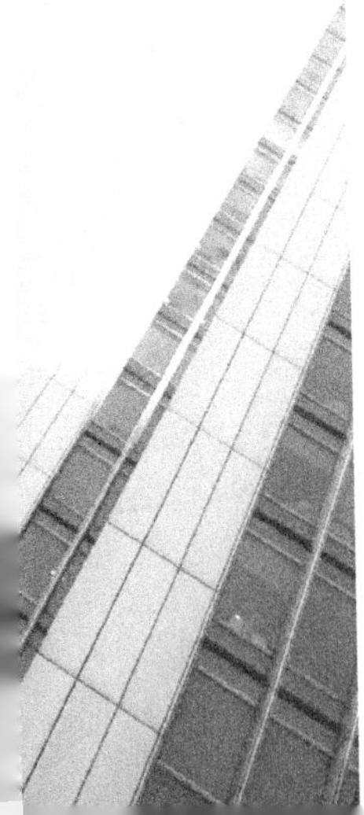

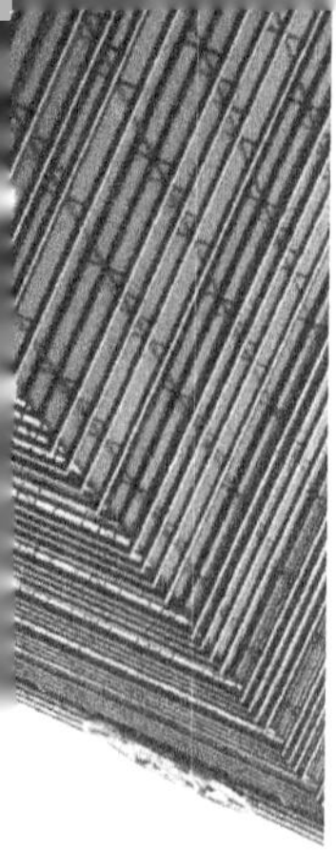

DAY 1:

11. What messages did I receive about love, safety, or success that no longer feel aligned?
12. What am I afraid to admit to myself?
13. What relationship patterns do I continue to repeat?
14. What is the cost of staying the same?
15. What do I believe about healing?
16. What fears surface when I imagine being truly healed?
17. What do I need to hear right now, and can I say it to myself?
18. How do I define accountability, and how am I practicing it?
19. Where do I feel stuck—and why?
20. What does my inner child still need from me?
21. What lies have I believed about who I am?
22. How has trauma shaped the way I protect myself?

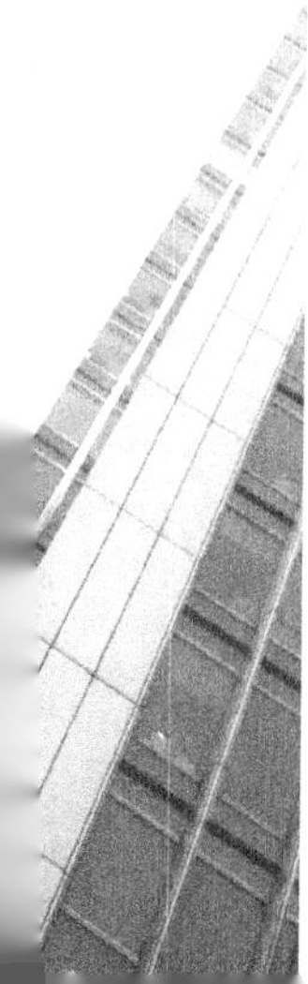

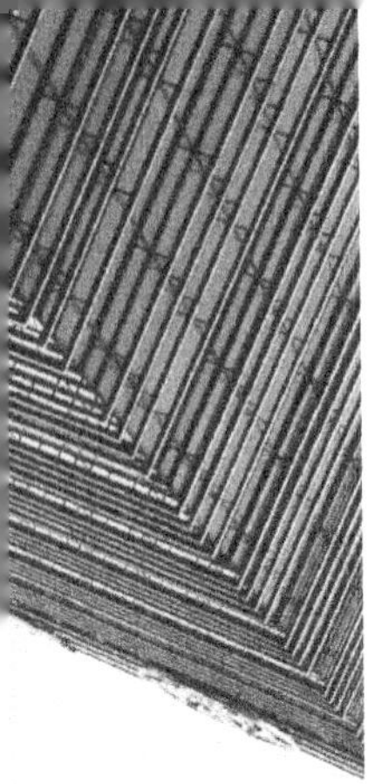

DAY 1:

23. What emotions do I avoid—and what would happen if I faced them?
24. How do I sabotage my own growth?
25. What patterns did I inherit from family or culture?
26. What am I afraid will happen if I let go of the past?
27. What boundaries do I need to strengthen?
28. Where do I need to be more honest with myself?
29. What parts of me have I abandoned to survive?
30. What would self-trust look like in action?
31. How do I react when I feel unseen or misunderstood?
32. What cycles am I being called to break?
33. What is my truth, and am I ready to live in it?

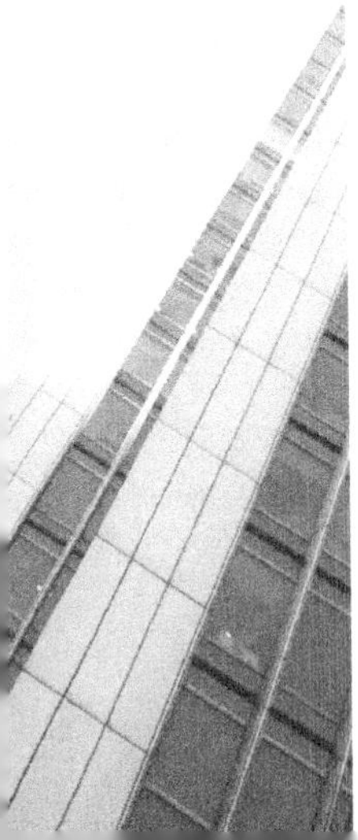

NOTES

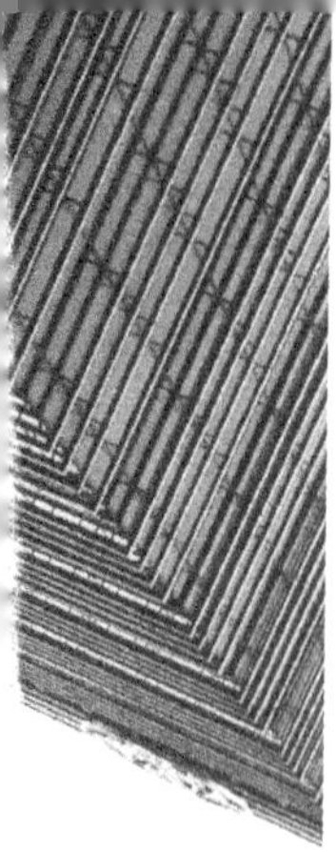

DAY 2:

Day 2: "Sealing the Cut, Invoking the Shift"

Theme: Letting Go, Forgiveness, and Bold Declaration

Definition:

This is the day of spiritual surgery—cutting cords, letting go of emotional baggage, forgiving what has lingered too long, and boldly declaring who you are becoming. It is sealing the wound with sacred fire and saying: "No more."

Why It Matters:

We carry too much. People, energy, guilt, anger, shame, fear. Letting go is not passive—it is intentional release. Forgiveness is the spiritual unlock that lets you rewrite your story and begin again. And bold declarations shift your timeline.

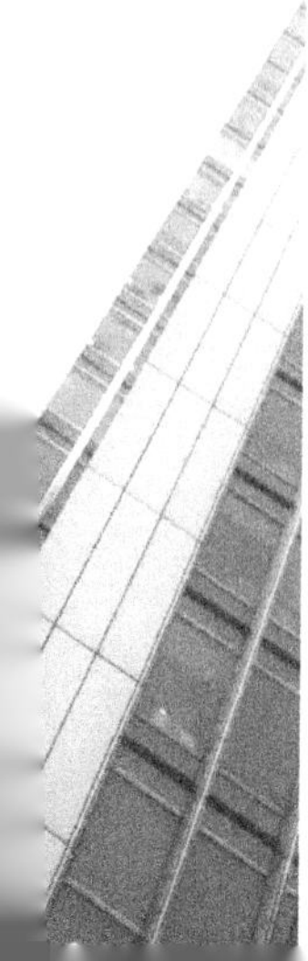

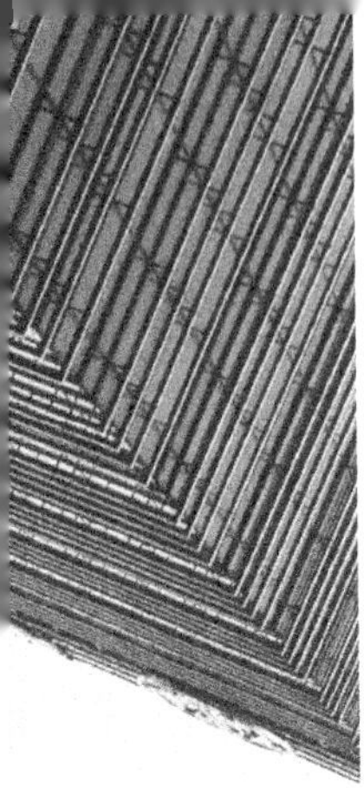

DAY 2:

Example:

You've been carrying resentment toward a parent for never showing up for you. You feared that forgiving them meant excusing them. But today, you realize forgiveness is for your freedom, not their comfort. You cut the energetic cord. You say aloud:

"I forgive. I let go. I choose peace. I am no longer tethered to this pain. I walk in wholeness."

"You are not just sealing wounds—you are opening gates."

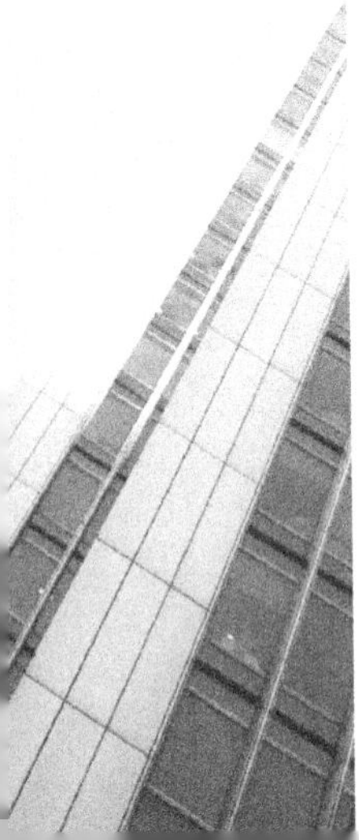

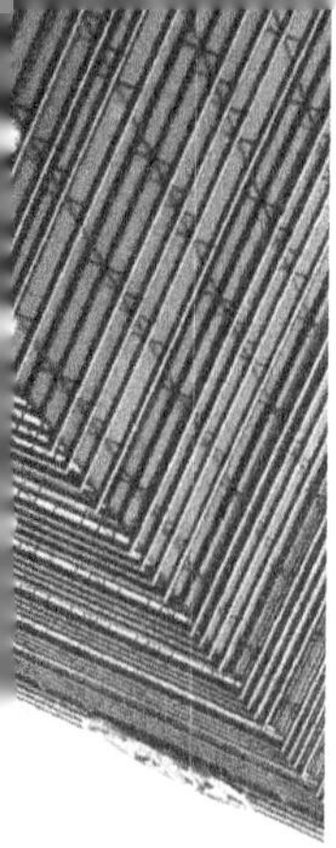

DAY 2:

Day 2: Sealing the Cut, Invoking the Shift

Theme: Letting Go, Forgiveness, and Bold Declaration
Focus: Cutting cords, self-forgiveness, spiritual protection, making a new declaration

Letting go is not always about weakness. Sometimes, it's the most courageous act of love. Day 2 is about choosing to cut ties—energetic, emotional, mental, spiritual—that keep you bound to stories, people, and pain that no longer serve your highest path.

Sealing the cut means more than walking away; it means spiritually and emotionally closing the chapter with intention. You are not abandoning the lessons, but releasing the weight.

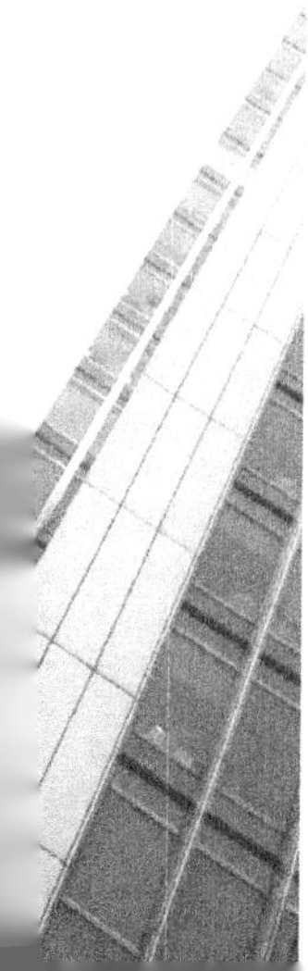

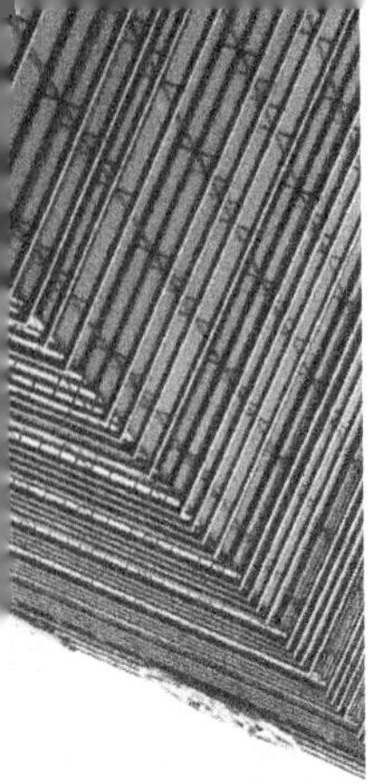

DAY 2:

You do not need to carry guilt, resentment, or obligation in order to honor your story. You are allowed to forgive. You are allowed to rewrite the narrative.

This day also calls for declaration: to invoke divine support, to speak new intentions out loud, to claim your path boldly. It's time to invite help from the unseen, from the divine, from your higher self. You don't have to do this alone.

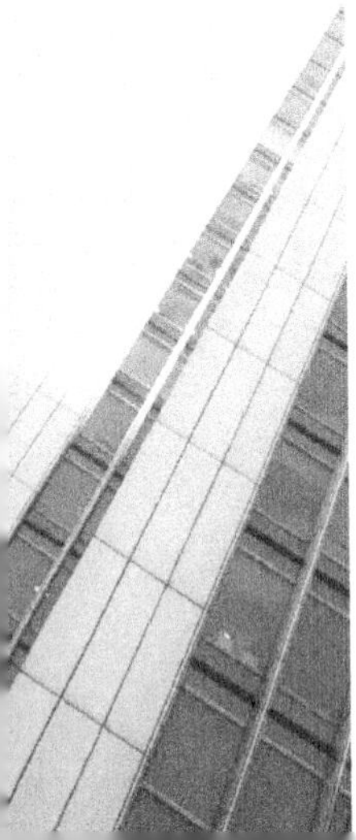

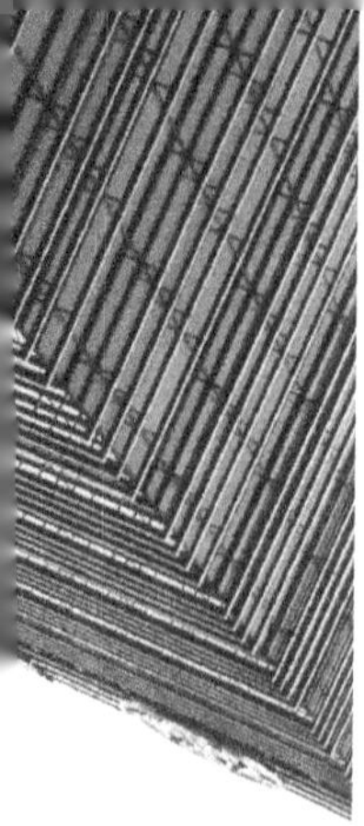

DAY 2:

CORD-CUTTING & SOUL HEALING

Definition in Real Time:

Cord-cutting is the energetic process of releasing unhealthy attachments, relationships, traumas, karmic cycles, and psychic entanglements that bind your energy to people, events, and patterns that no longer serve your growth or your truth.

This is not just a ritual of "letting go" in the mind. This is an intentional act of spiritual surgery—uprooting the entire tree, not just clipping the branches.

It's about removing energetic debris and soul ties that act as anchors, keeping you emotionally and spiritually stagnant.

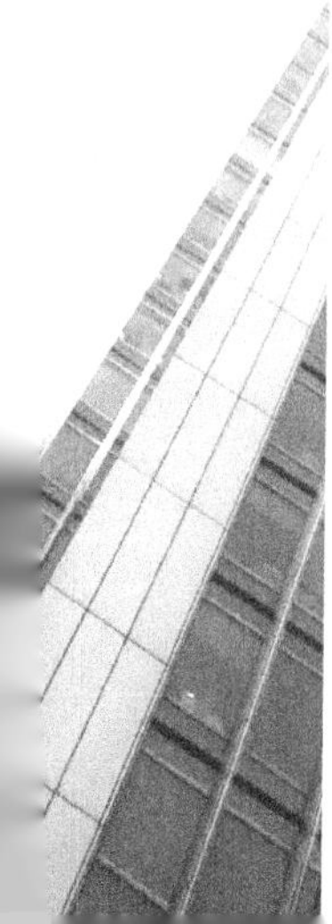

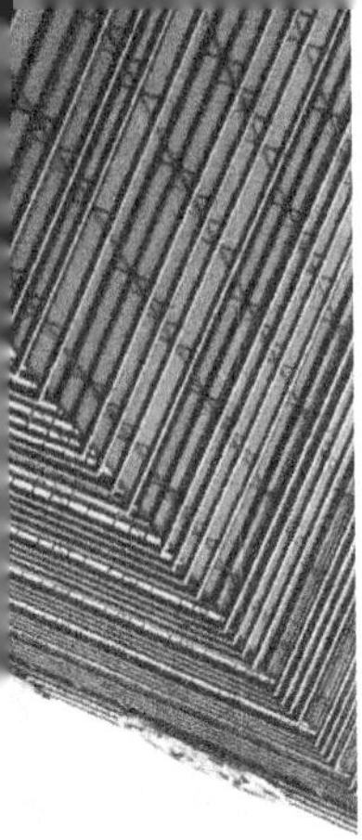

DAY 2:

Soul healing is the sacred repair and realignment of your spiritual core. It is the reawakening of the inner you—the part of you that existed before the trauma, the grief, the betrayal.

Many walk through life with a vacant spirit, doing but not being, breathing but not living. Soul healing is the process of coming back home to yourself.

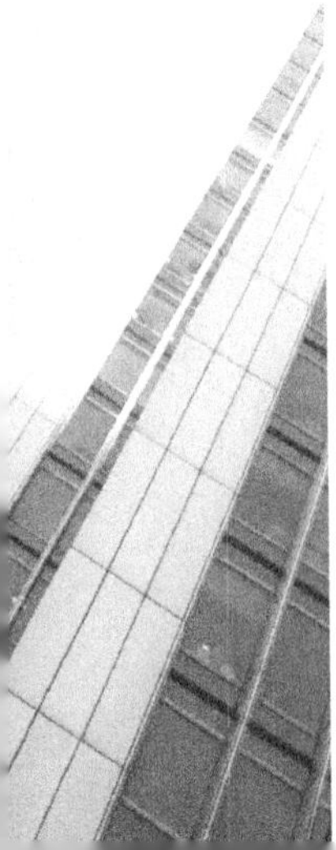

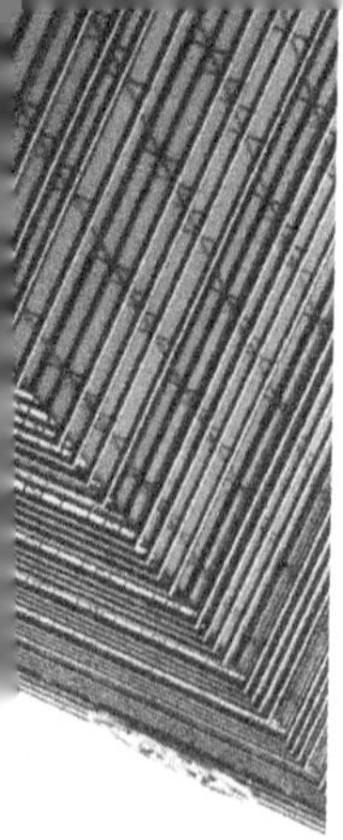

DAY 2:

Why It's Crucial:

- You cannot walk into your new story while holding onto the dust and dirt of the old one.
- Uncut cords drain your power—you give your energy away to people who are no longer present, or to experiences that are no longer real but still rule your emotions.
- Spiritual parasites feed on old cords—this is how emotional toxicity and spiritual bondage continue generation after generation.
- Soul healing allows you to restore the fragmented pieces of your spirit. Without this, life can feel numb, shallow, and without purpose.

"You are not stuck. You're entangled. It's time to untangle, release, and return to your original design."

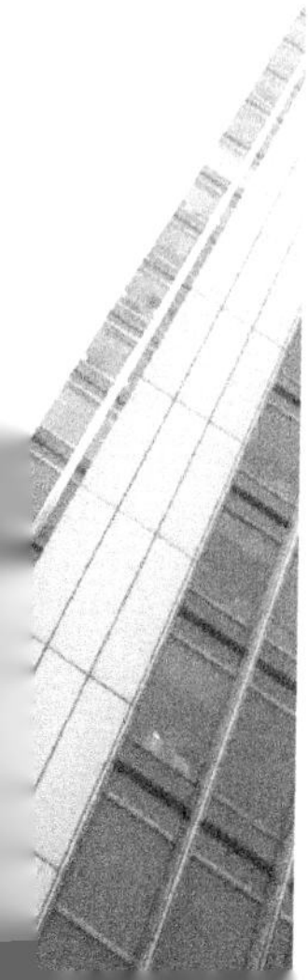

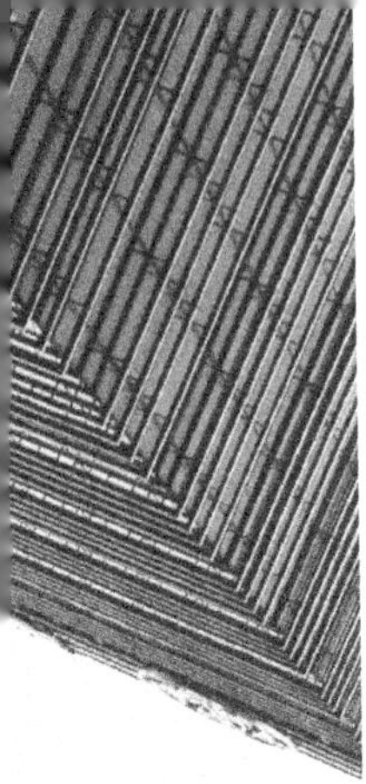

DAY 2:

DIVINE HELP & ANGELIC ASSISTANCE

Definition in Real Time:

Divine help and angelic assistance are the supernatural interventions and spiritual presences that guide, support, protect, and uplift us beyond what we can do in the flesh alone.

These forces—ancestors, angels, spirit guides, divine beings—are always around, always waiting for your permission to step in.

This is not fantasy—it is energy. It is projection. Divine beings don't always enter your body; they often project their frequency onto your aura, influencing your thoughts, nudging your steps, aligning your path with unseen grace.

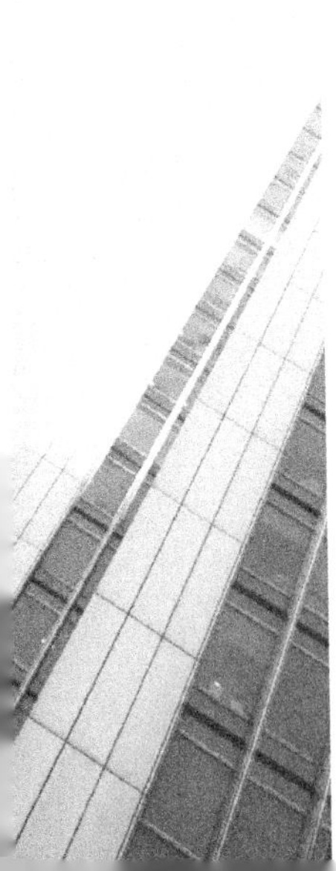

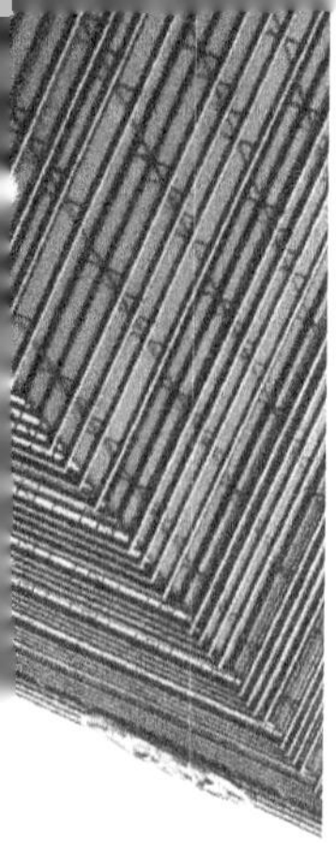

DAY 2:

Negativity works the same way—it doesn't always enter, it projects. But many people internalize projected darkness, mistaking it for identity. When we learn the power of our own projection and the assistance of higher energies, we rise above fear.

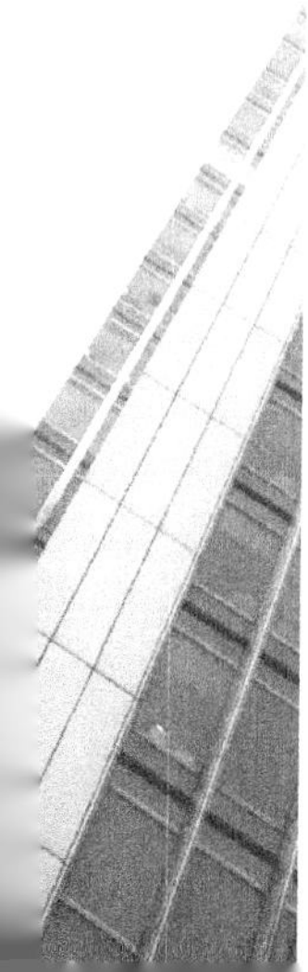

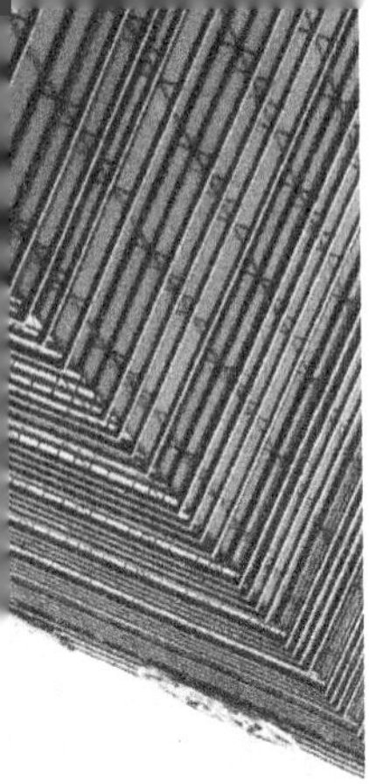

DAY 2:

Why It's Crucial:

- Help is always available, but spiritual law honors free will. You must ask.
- You are not meant to heal or carry the burden alone. Divine help is what moves the mountain when your strength is gone.
- It reminds you that you are never alone. Every step is witnessed, and every prayer is heard—even the silent ones.

"Heaven is not far—it is frequency. Change yours, and you'll hear them."

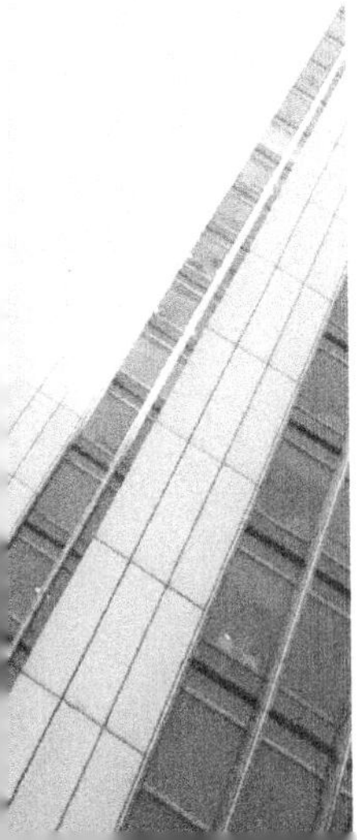

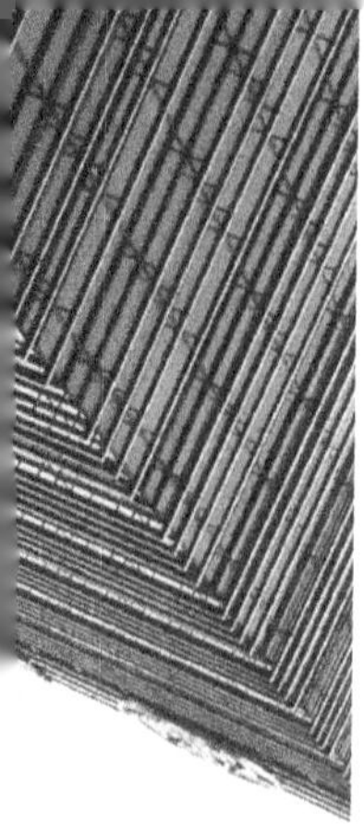

DAY 2:

Prayer for Cord-Cutting and Soul Healing

Divine Presence,

I call on your light to sever every tie that holds me back from my freedom. Cut the cords that drain my energy and keep me repeating the same patterns.

Release me from the attachments that no longer align with my highest truth.

Heal the spaces those ties once filled—fill them with peace, love, and divine clarity.

Let no wound be left open, no space be left void. I do not wish to carry fragments of the past with me into my future.

Where I once clung to pain, replace it with peace.

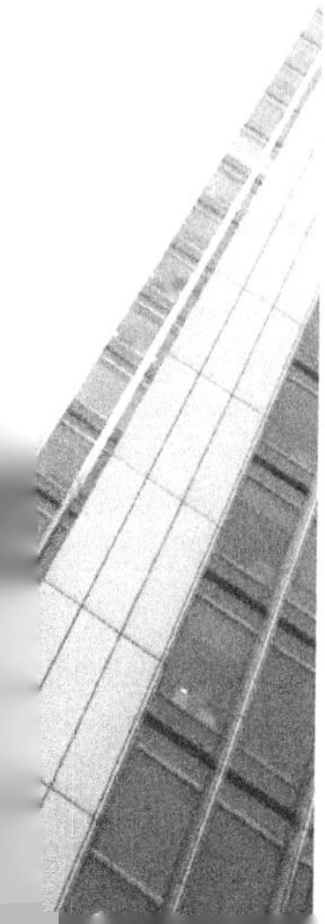

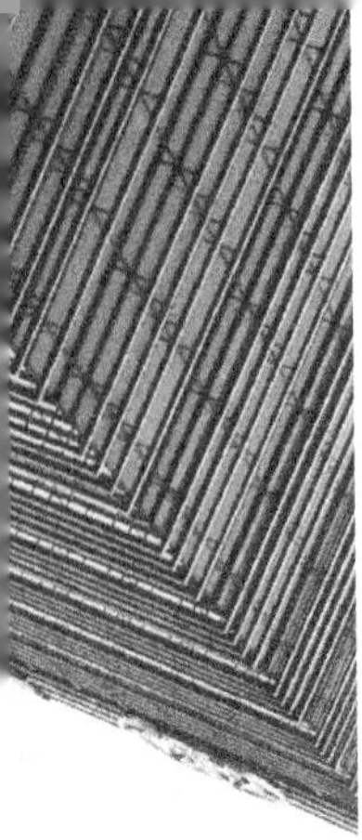

DAY 2:

Where I once needed validation, remind me of my worth.

Where I once feared being alone, anchor me in divine companionship.

Seal every cut with grace. I move forward in wholeness and truth.

Amen.

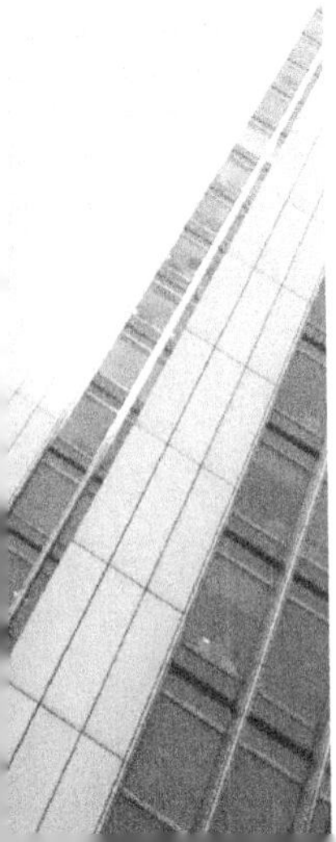

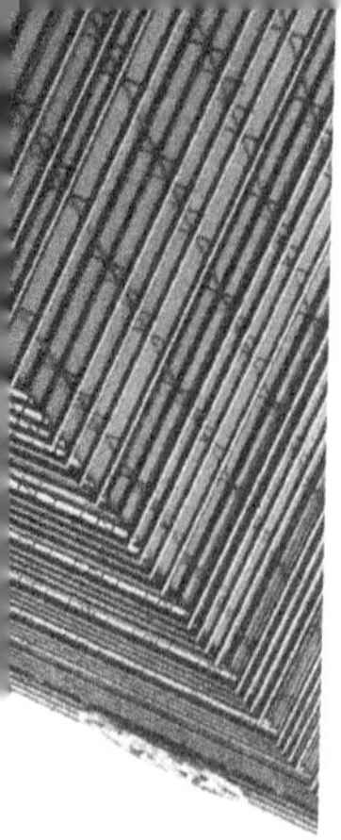

DAY 2:

Prayer to Invoke Divine Help and Angelic Assistance

Beloved Divine,

I acknowledge that I am in need of help beyond my own strength. I no longer try to carry it all alone. I welcome the support of divine guides, angels, ancestors, and protectors who walk in light and love.

Send me clarity when I feel lost.
Send me signs when I need reassurance.
Send me strength when I feel weak.

Surround me with divine protection as I make this shift in my spirit.

I open my heart to receive help. I surrender the need to control every outcome. I ask for guidance and accept it with humility.

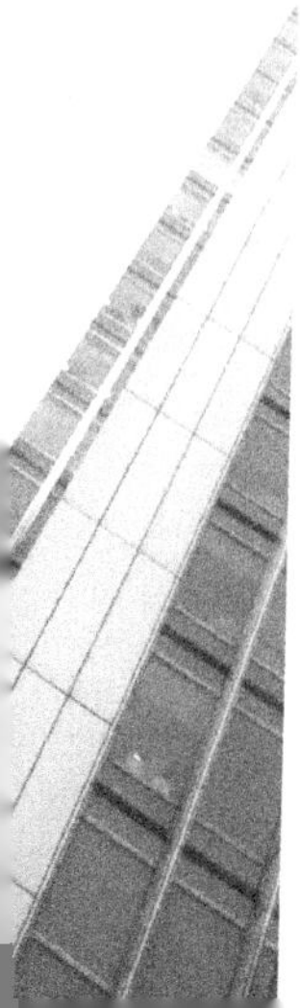

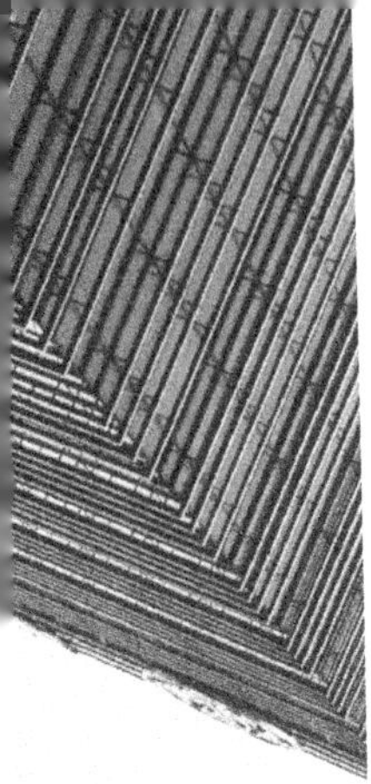

DAY 2:

Let your presence go before me. Let your love wrap around me.

With every step I take, may I feel that I am not alone.

Amen.

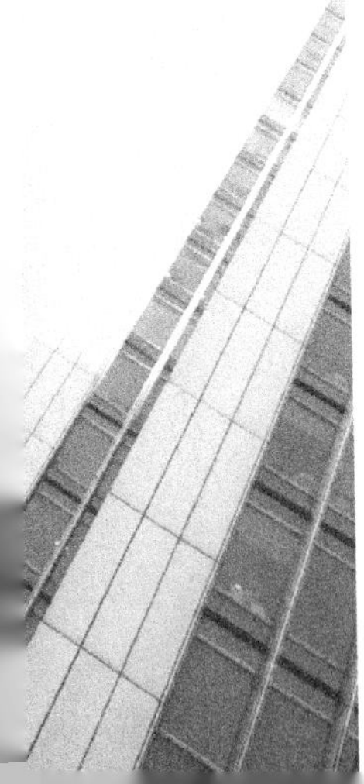

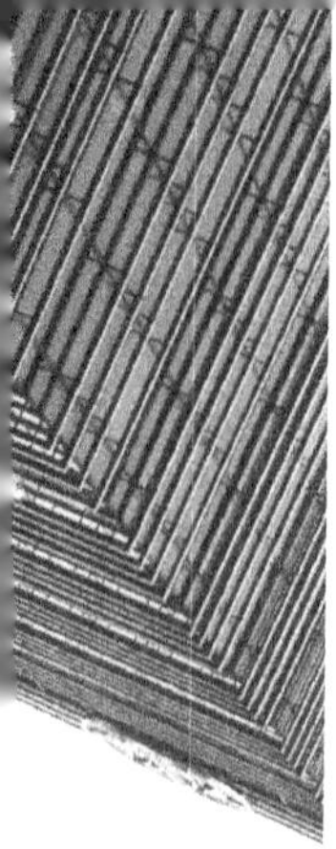

DAY 2:

FORGIVENESS & REWRITING THE STORY

Definition in Real Time:

Forgiveness is the conscious, spiritual act of releasing your inner prison, not excusing wrongs but removing their power over your peace.

It is the refusal to let pain become your identity. It is a self-liberation.

Rewriting your story is the sacred act of reclaiming authorship of your life. It's choosing to become the narrator, not the victim.

It's where healing becomes creation. You shift the narrative from "what happened to me" to "what I now choose to create from it."

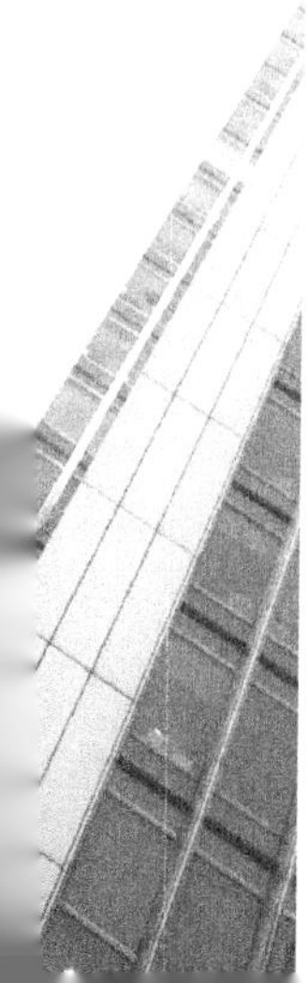

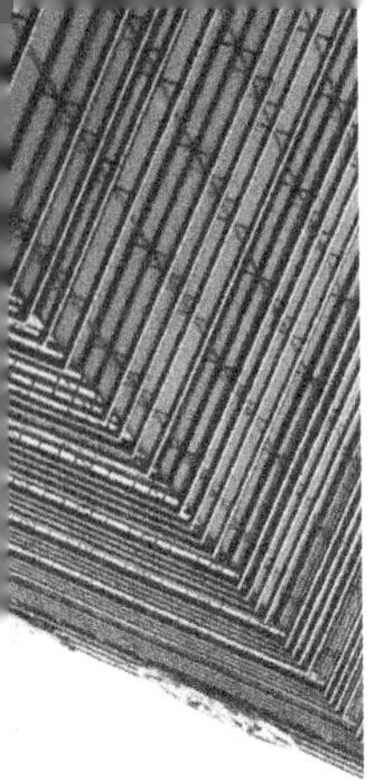

DAY 2:

Too many hold on to unforgiveness as if it gives them power, as if staying angry proves something. But unforgiveness is an energy leak. It rots the container from the inside out. Forgiveness is not about the other person—it's about your own rebirth.

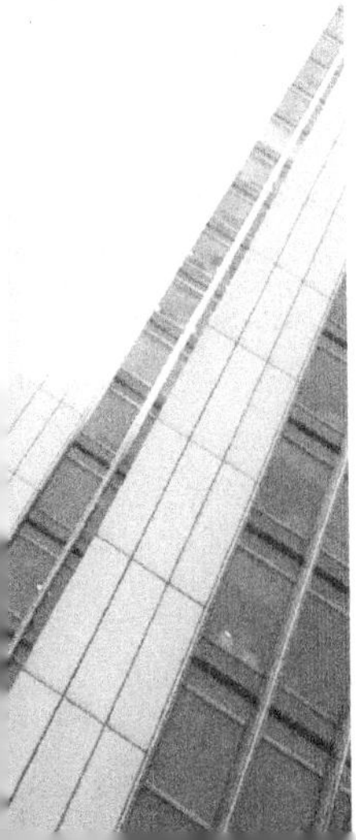

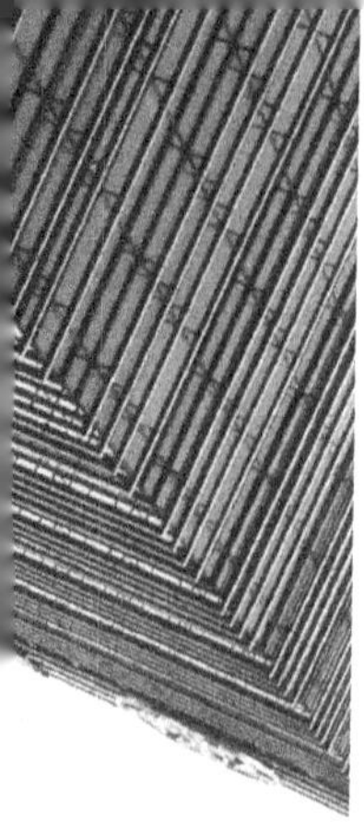

DAY 2:

Why It's Crucial:

- Bitterness blinds you. Forgiveness clears the vision.
- Holding on burns your energy and blocks your blessings.
- Rewriting your story allows you to activate your voice, your truth, your divine spark—and craft a life beyond the wounds.

"Your past is a chapter, not your name. Rewrite it. You are the pen. You are the power."

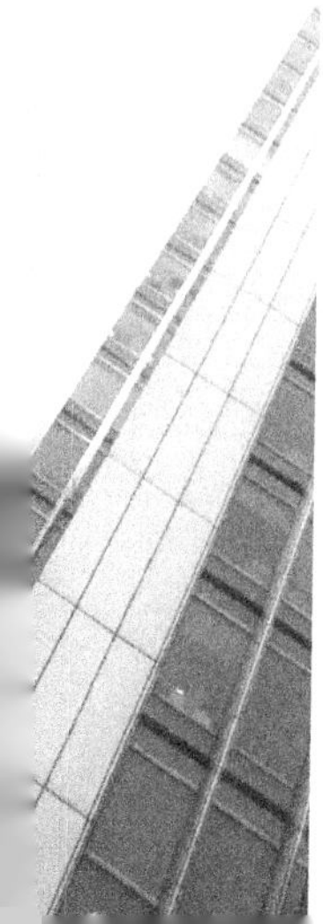

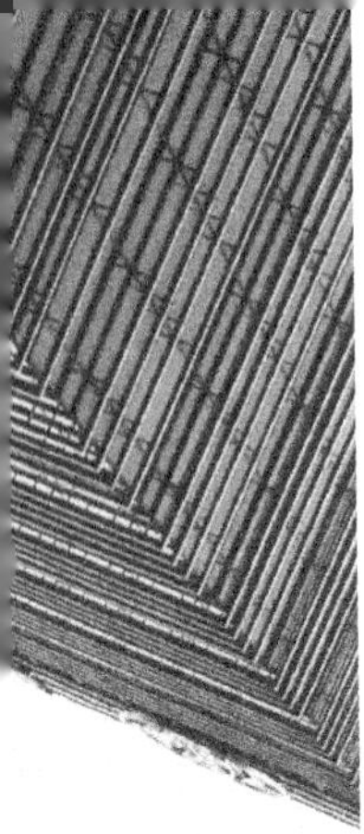

DAY 2:

Final Reflections:

Letting go is not a soft process—it is spiritual warfare.

Cord-cutting is exorcism of the invisible chains.

Soul healing is resurrection.
Divine help is a whisper away.

Forgiveness is release.
And rewriting is revolution.

"This day is not about letting go for the sake of peace. It's about letting go because peace is your birthright. Because you are no longer available for what dims your light."

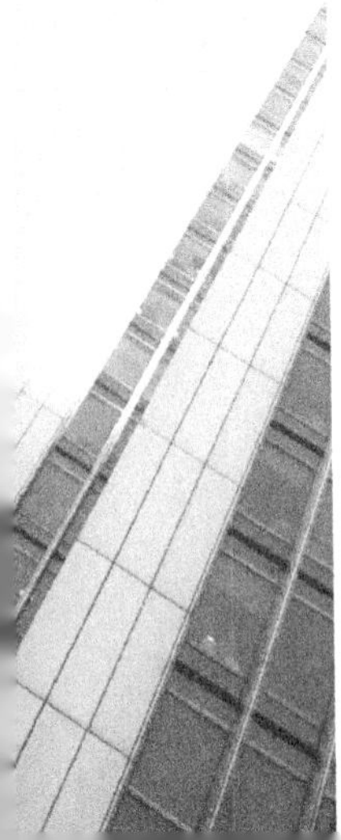

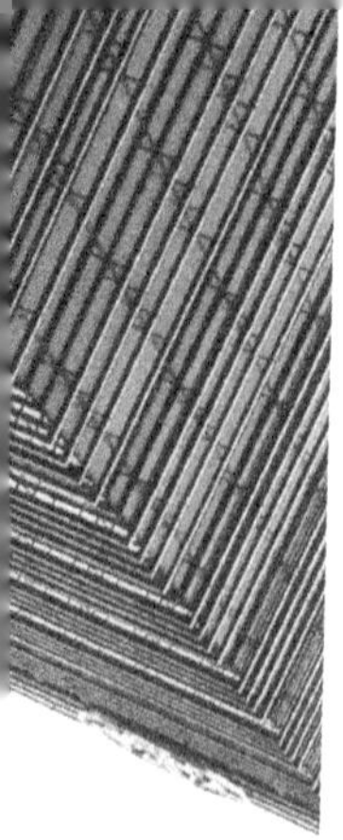

DAY 2:

Prayer for Forgiveness and Rewriting the Story

Sacred Spirit,

I come to you ready to forgive—not because I condone the pain, but because I am choosing to be free.

I forgive those who hurt me, knowingly or unknowingly. I release the need to hold onto the pain as proof of my strength.

I forgive myself for every time I betrayed my own voice, for every decision made from fear, for every version of me who did not know better.
I am not my shame. I am not my regrets.

I am a soul who is learning and unlearning, healing and evolving.

Help me rewrite my story.

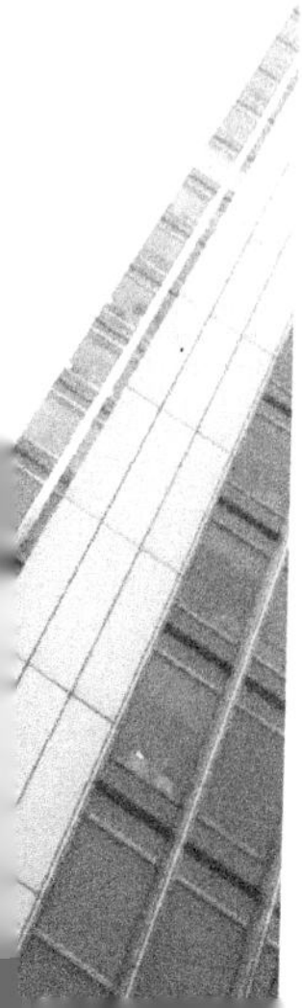

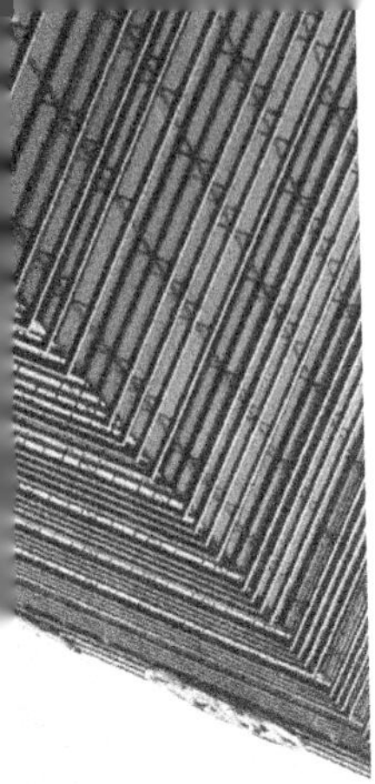

DAY 2:

Let it no longer be shaped by victimhood, but by victory.

Let it reflect wisdom, not just wounds.
Let it rise from grace, not guilt.
I reclaim authorship over my life.

My story begins again—here, now, today.

Amen.

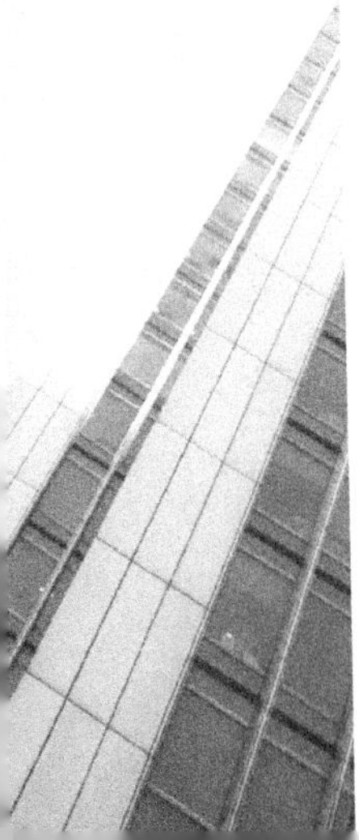

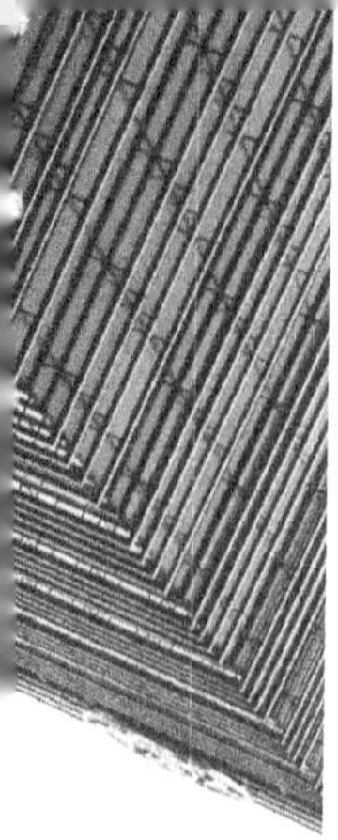

DAY 2:

33 Affirmations for Day 2

1. I forgive myself for not knowing better.
2. I am open to divine help.
3. My voice is powerful and sacred.
4. I cut all energetic cords that no longer serve me.
5. I am free to choose a new story.
6. I accept myself fully, including my past.
7. I welcome protection and peace.
8. I allow myself to release without fear.
9. I am not defined by old versions of me.
10. I speak healing into my timeline.
11. I am supported by the divine in every step.
12. My past does not hold power over me.
13. I allow myself to move forward in grace.
14. I trust my higher path.

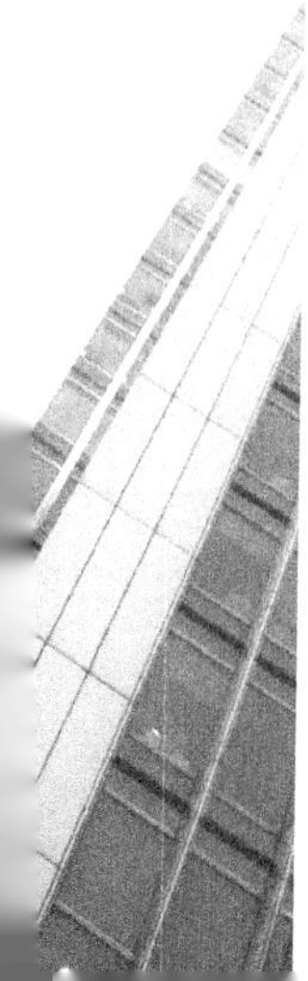

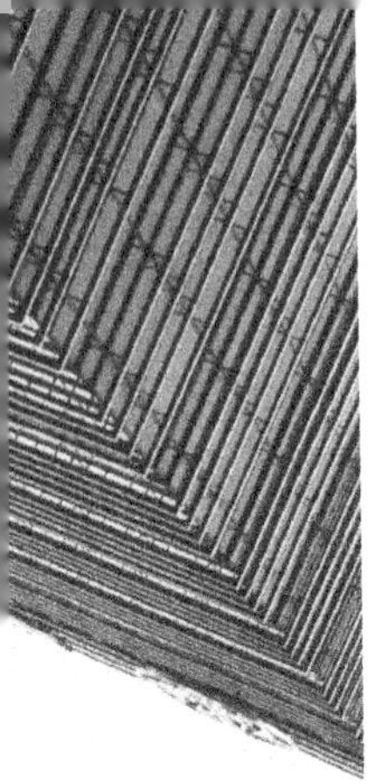

DAY 2:

15. I release shame and guilt.
16. I believe in the power of renewal.
17. I am not alone in my healing journey.
18. I give myself permission to forgive.
19. I trust the guidance of my spirit.
20. I invite angels and guides to walk with me.
21. I am a new creation with every breath.
22. I no longer hold on to what is no longer mine.
23. I am worthy of beginning again.
24. I allow joy to return.
25. I am energetically protected and grounded.
26. I am guided by divine wisdom.
27. I am gentle with myself as I grow.
28. I welcome closure and peace.
29. I am rewriting my story in alignment with truth.
30. I am no longer bound by pain.
31. I choose love, power, and clarity.
32. I am no longer attached to outcomes.
33. I forgive to free myself.

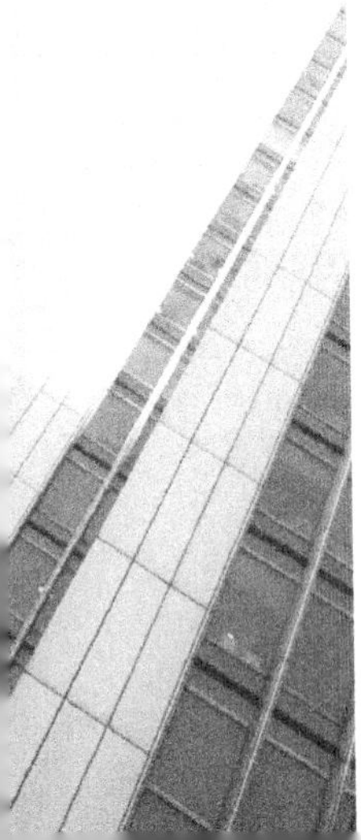

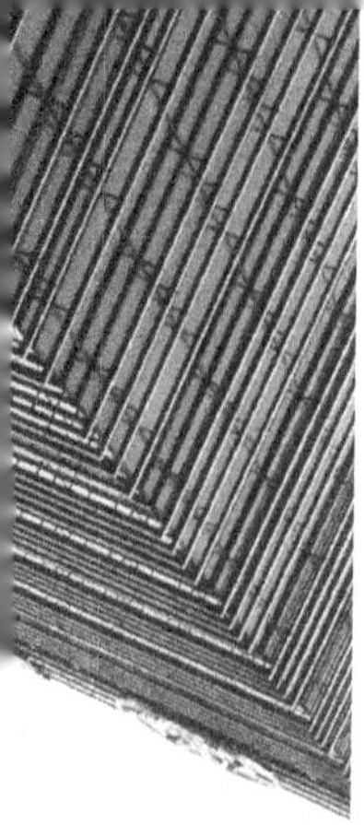

DAY 2:

33 Deep Questions for Reflection and Journaling

1. What am I afraid to release, and why?
2. What forgiveness do I still withhold—from myself or others?
3. If I believed the divine was with me now, what would I boldly declare?
4. Who or what am I still energetically tied to, and how is that affecting my life?
5. What stories about myself do I keep repeating?
6. What would forgiveness look like in action for me?
7. What do I gain by holding onto resentment?
8. What pain am I still using as identity?
9. What truth am I afraid to accept because of what it will require me to change?

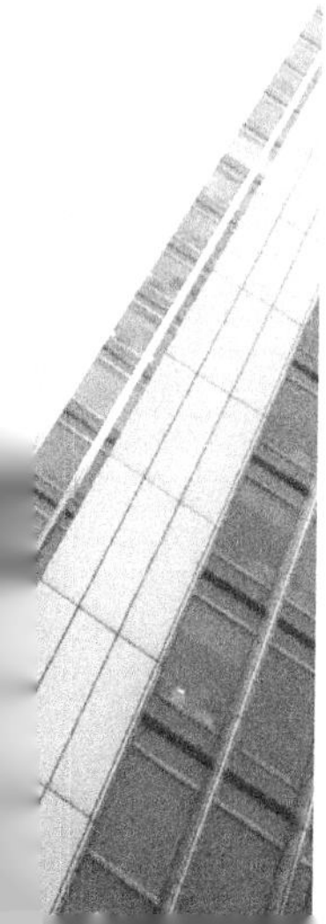

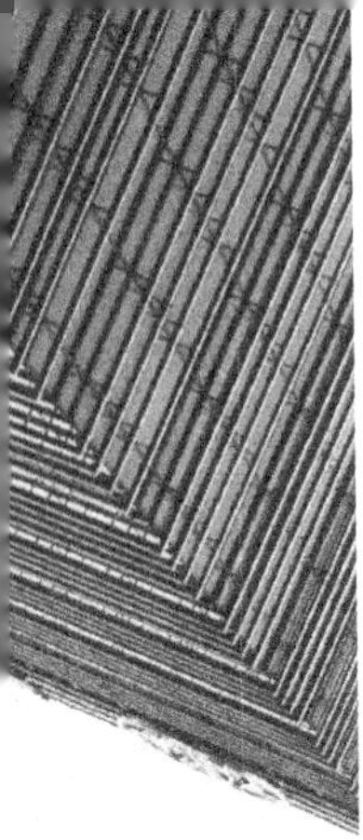

DAY 2:

10. When was the last time I forgave myself—and truly meant it?
11. What emotions do I experience when I consider cutting ties or walking away?
12. What boundaries do I need to reinforce to protect my peace?
13. In what areas of my life do I need divine help right now?
14. Where am I refusing support, and why?
15. What do I believe about asking for help?
16. How have I been rewriting or reshaping my story recently?
17. What version of my story am I ready to retire?
18. What parts of my past still feel "unfinished," and what do they need?
19. What would my healed self say to the person I used to be?
20. What have I internalized that was never truly mine to carry?

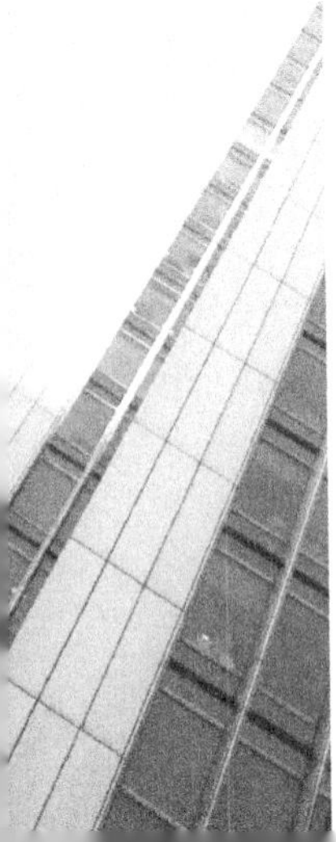

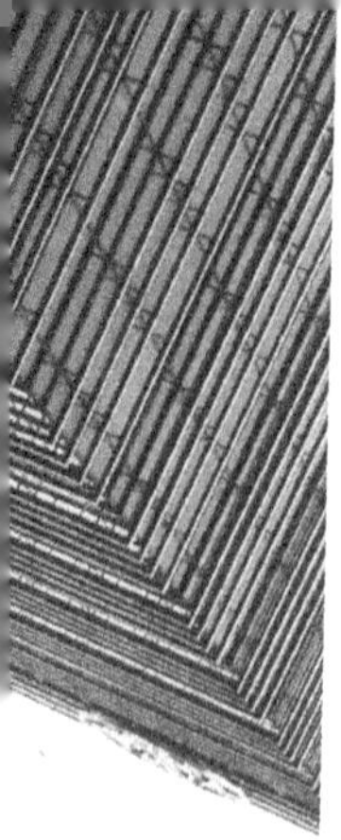

DAY 2:

21. Who or what drains my energy the most?
22. How do I know when I've forgiven someone?
23. What guilt or shame do I still carry?
24. How would my life change if I released it?
25. What keeps me from fully forgiving myself?
26. What divine or spiritual forces do I feel most connected to, and why?
27. When do I feel most protected and supported?
28. How has my definition of forgiveness changed over time?
29. What am I being asked to say out loud and claim?
30. What is one truth I am afraid to speak, but ready to own?
31. What spiritual practices help me feel safe and anchored?
32. What symbolic act could I do to mark this shift in me?
33. What do I declare over my life moving forward?

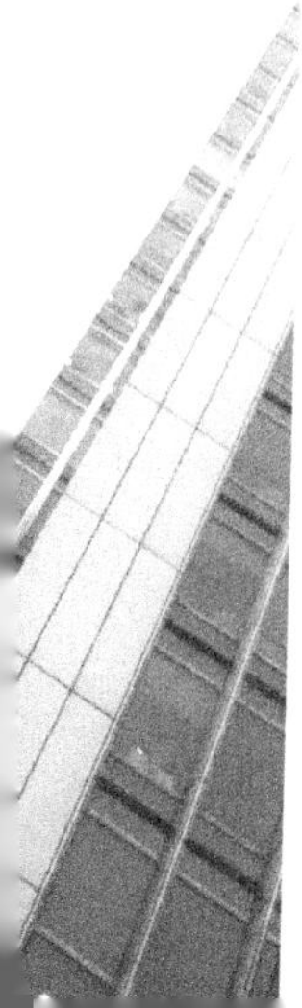

NOTES

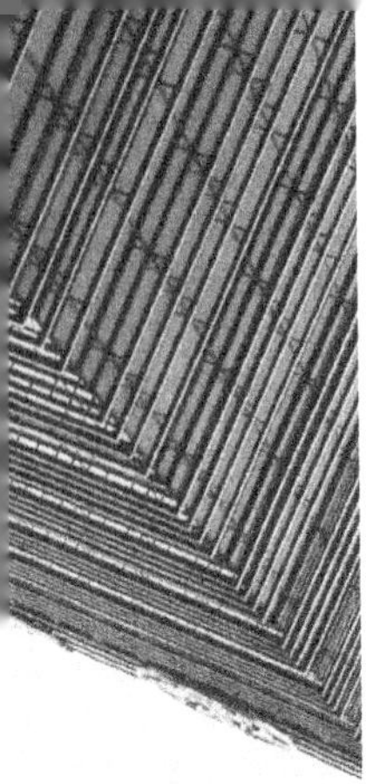

DAY 3:

Day 3: "Gratitude and Knowing"
Theme: Gratitude, Trust, and Rebirth

Definition:

After reflection and release comes renewal. This day is about rising with gratitude, building trust in the divine process, and rebirthing your energy.

It's recognizing what is working, what has protected you, and what you are growing into. It's stepping into the now with reverence and faith.

Why It Matters:

Gratitude realigns your frequency. Trust expands your vision. Rebirth begins with the awareness that you are already becoming.

You've cleared the field—now you plant the seed.

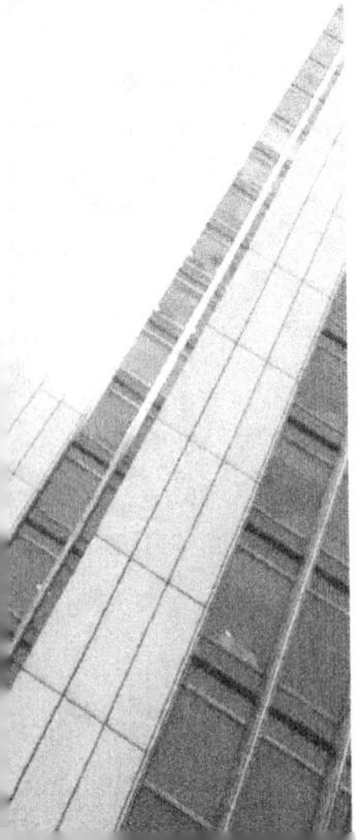

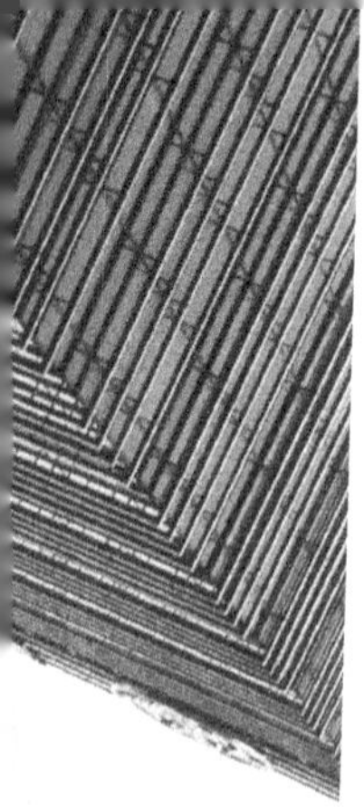

DAY 3:

Example:

After cutting cords with toxic past relationships, you feel empty but free. Instead of mourning the loss, you say:

“Thank you for the lesson. Thank you for this breath. Thank you for the space to receive what is mine.”

You trust that what is meant for you is flowing toward you now. You walk with new eyes.

“Gratitude is the song of rebirth. It says: I see now. I trust now. I rise now.”

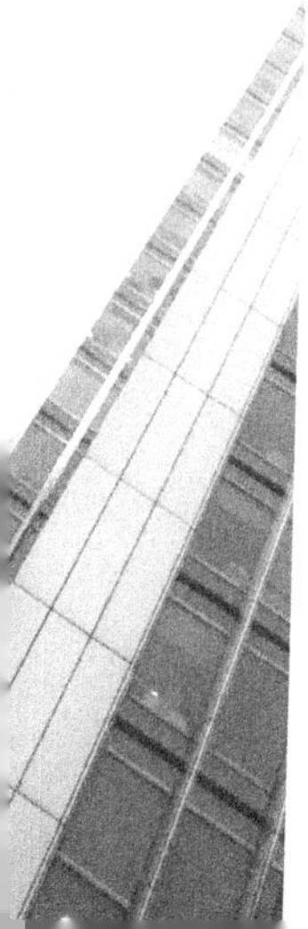

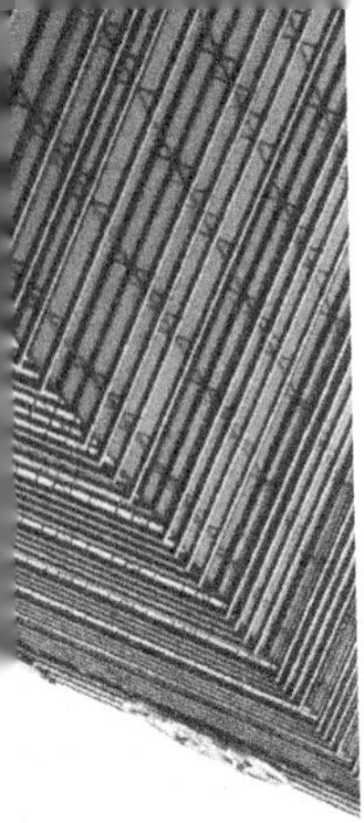

DAY 3:

Day 3: "Gratitude and Knowing"

Theme: Gratitude, Trust, and Rebirth
Focus: Owning your healing, giving thanks, walking forward in certainty

Definition of the Theme:

This day marks the completion of a sacred inner cycle. You have reflected. You have released. Now, you rise.

This is the day of divine awareness—a deep exhale, a clear sky after a storm. Gratitude is more than being thankful—it is the spiritual key that unlocks peace, attracts blessings, and realigns you with the truth of who you are.

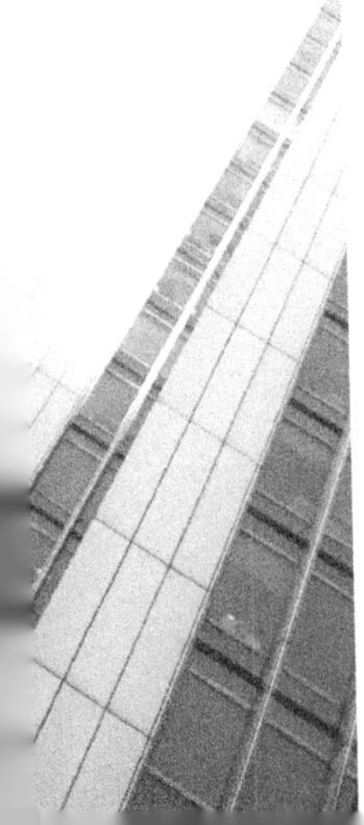

Trust is not about certainty in outcomes—it is certainty in Source. It is choosing to walk in the knowing, even before you see the full manifestation. Rebirth isn't always loud. Sometimes it's the quiet confidence that says, "I know who I am now."

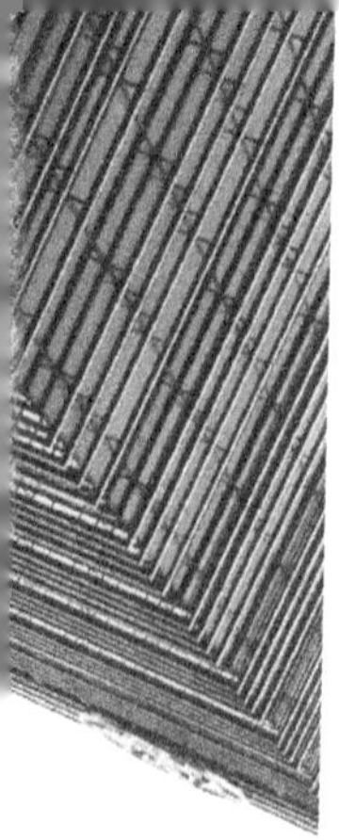

DAY 3:

1. Prayer of Thanksgiving for the Shift

"There is nothing you can reach, get, or hold unless you're grateful."

Purpose: Gratitude multiplies miracles. This prayer honors the journey and activates abundance by recognizing the shift that has already taken place.

Example:

"Thank you for every closed door that protected me. Thank you for every truth revealed. Thank you for what has left, and thank you for what is now arriving. I honor the shift in my soul."

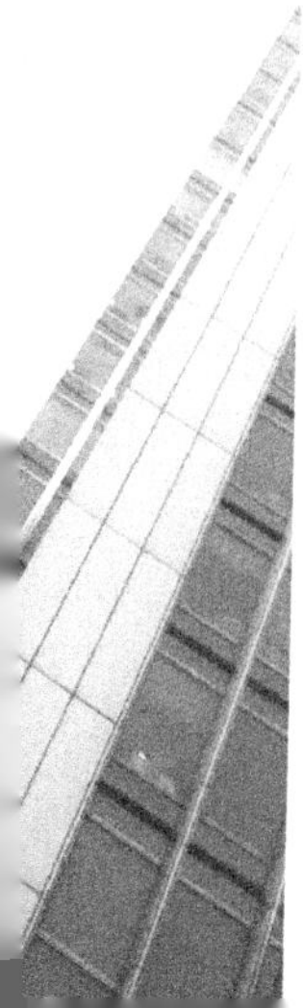

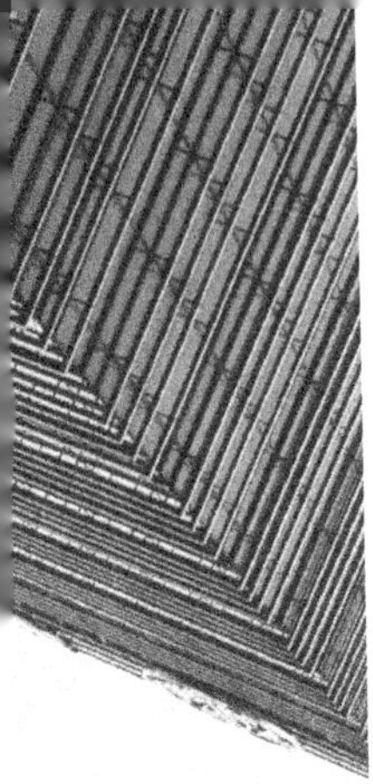

DAY 3:

2. Prayer of Celebration and Confidence

"Celebrate yourself before waiting for the world to clap."

Purpose: To declare your worth, celebrate your becoming, and stand tall in your sacred confidence.

Example:

"Today, I celebrate myself. I honor my power, my effort, my truth. I will not wait for outside validation—I am already chosen, already worthy, already divine."

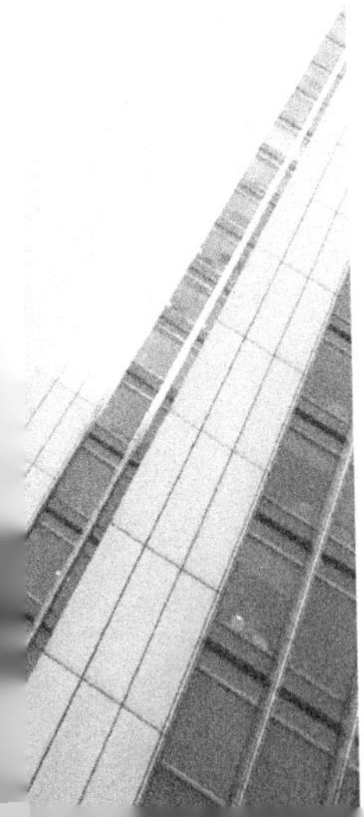

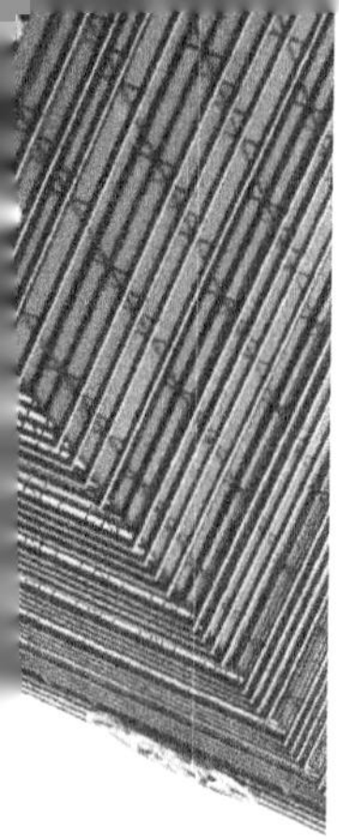

DAY 3:

3. Prayer to Walk in Alignment with Peace

“Nothing can thrive without peace and alignment.”

Purpose: To move forward with inner harmony, grounded in clarity and spirit-led direction. This is a prayer for true alignment with purpose, body, soul, and spirit.

Example:

"Guide me in peace. Align my steps with your light. Where there is chaos, restore calm. Where there is confusion, bring order. Let my every step echo wholeness."

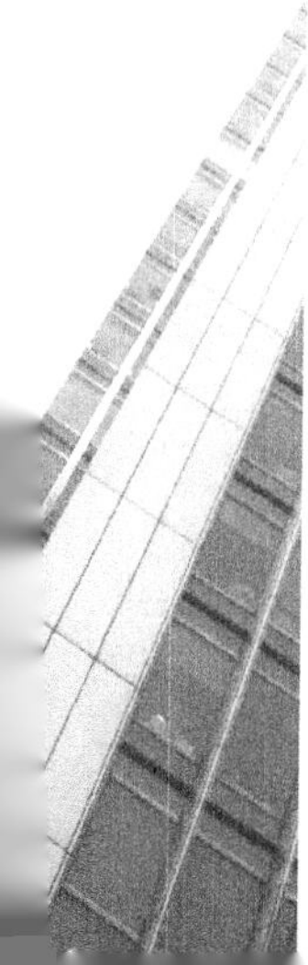

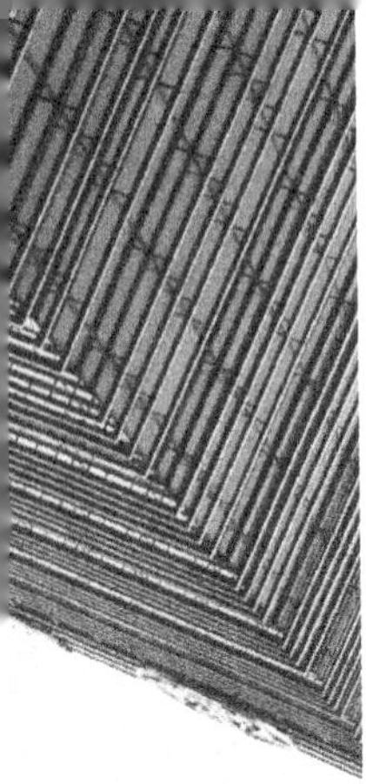

DAY 3:

33 Affirmations

1. I walk in the knowing, not just the hoping.
2. It is already done.
3. My life is divinely guided and renewed.
4. I trust the divine timing of my life.
5. I release fear and embrace flow.
6. I am enough as I am.
7. Peace is my home and my frequency.
8. I am no longer waiting—I am walking.
9. My past does not define my next.
10. I am worthy of softness and celebration.
11. Confidence lives in me now.
12. I move with ease and trust.
13. My gratitude opens new doors.
14. I have survived. I have grown. I have risen.
15. I celebrate my growth, even the silent parts.

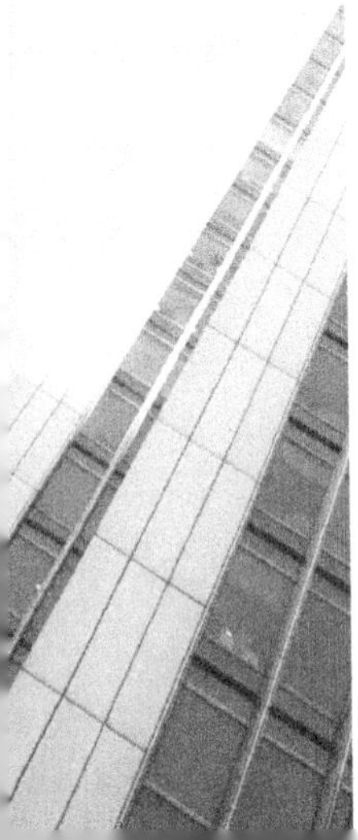

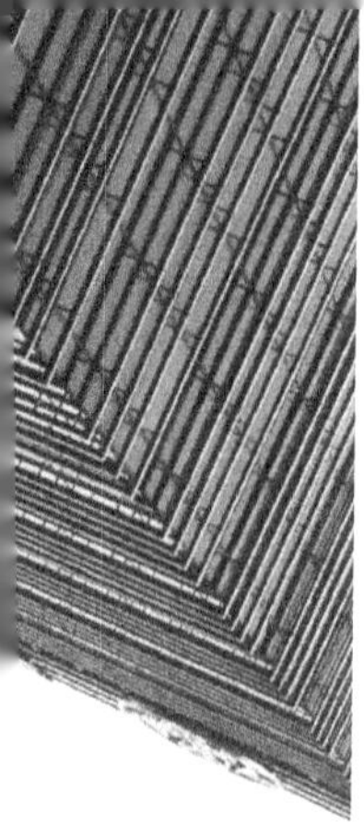

DAY 3:

16. Every breath is a new beginning.
17. I am the answered prayer of my ancestors.
18. Clarity flows to me effortlessly.
19. I trust the next chapter because I am the author.
20. I breathe in calm and exhale fear.
21. Divine alignment surrounds me.
22. I am protected and powered by grace.
23. My knowing is stronger than my doubt.
24. I am a vessel of peace and purpose.
25. I am reborn in this moment.
26. My spirit is steady, my heart is light.
27. I carry only what blesses me.
28. I rise with purpose and pride.
29. I trust my journey completely.
30. My healing is my strength.
31. I move in sacred confidence.
32. I celebrate myself daily.
33. I am home in myself. I am home to myself. I am home with myself.

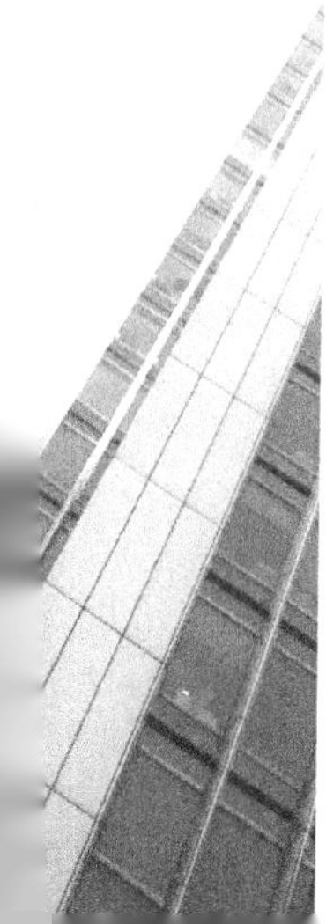

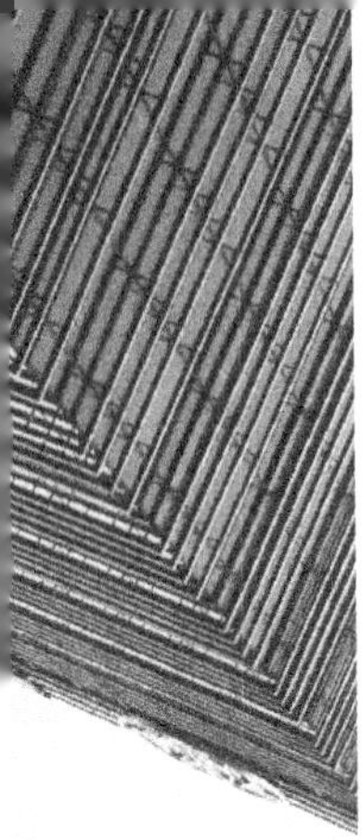

DAY 3:

33 Deep Questions (Journal Prompts)

1. What do I now know for sure?
2. What has changed within me over these three days?
3. What am I ready to build now that the weight is gone?
4. How has my definition of healing evolved?
5. What does peace now mean to me?
6. Where can I celebrate myself more often?
7. What am I no longer tolerating?
8. What energy do I want to bring into every room I enter?
9. What have I been afraid to trust, and why?
10. Who am I without the pain I carried?
11. How do I embody gratitude today?
12. What does confidence look like for me now?
13. What are the daily habits that align me with peace?
14. How has forgiveness freed me?

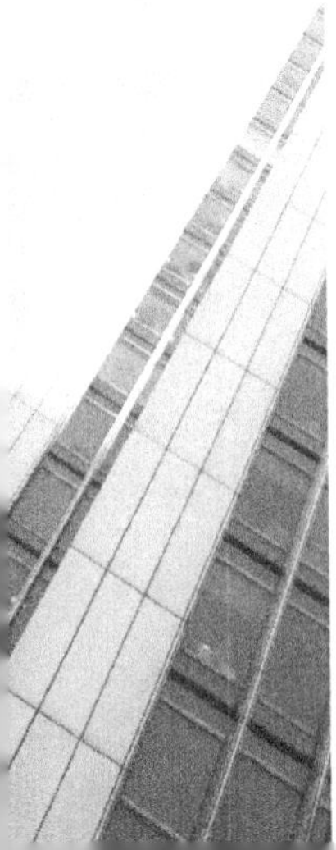

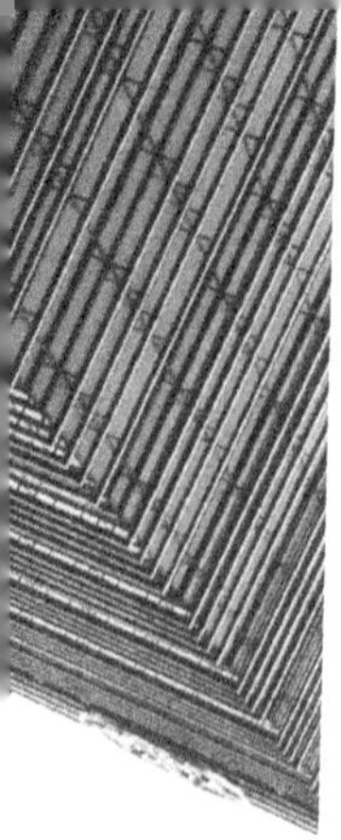

DAY 3:

15. What truth have I reclaimed?
16. What is my new declaration moving forward?
17. What role does my intuition play now?
18. What am I still holding back, and why?
19. How can I deepen my spiritual connection from this point?
20. Where do I feel reborn in my life?
21. What was the most powerful moment of this journey?
22. Who am I becoming now?
23. What fears have I proven wrong?
24. What blessings am I now ready to receive?
25. How will I honor my new chapter?
26. What does divine timing look like in my life?
27. How do I speak to myself now versus before?
28. What is no longer part of my identity?

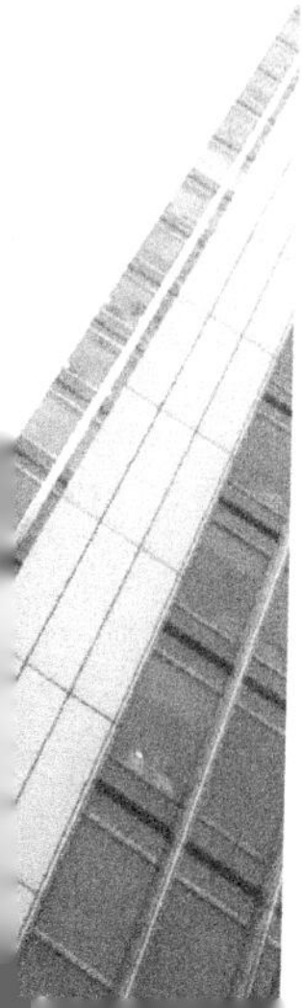

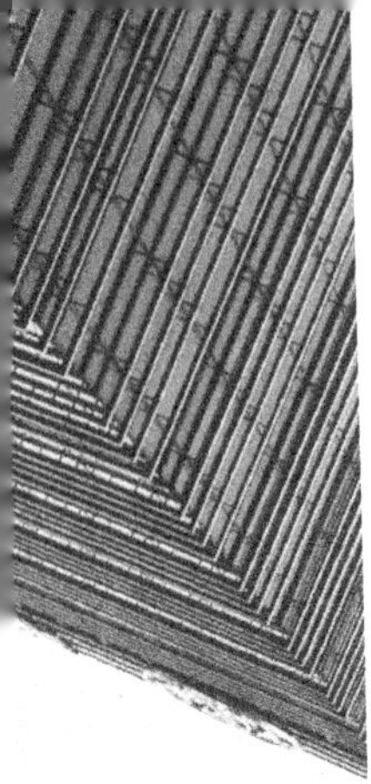

DAY 3:

29. How can I remain grounded in this knowing?
30. What am I now grateful for that I once resisted?
31. What is now clear to me that wasn't before?
32. How has trust been built or rebuilt in me?
33. How do I carry this shift with me beyond these three days?

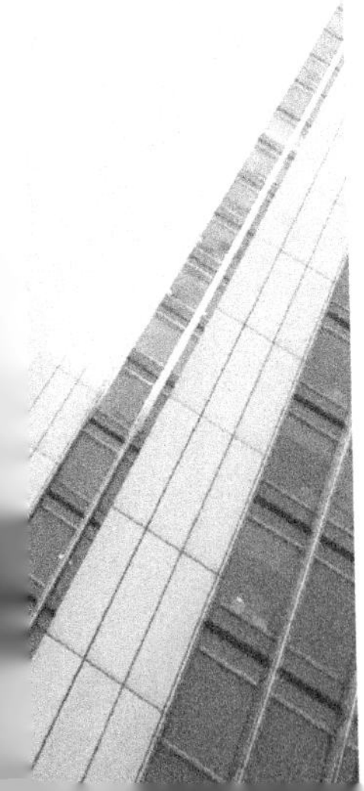

NOTES

[redacted]

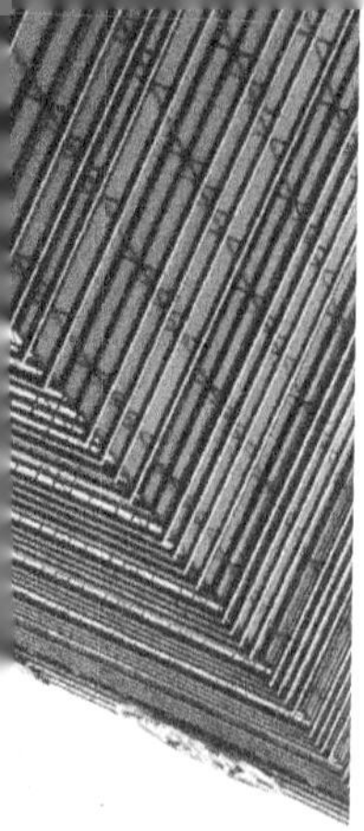

AFTER THE FAST:

AFTER THE FAST: Moving Forward in Power

You've completed the 3-day fast. What now?

You've walked through reflection, release, and rebirth. You've acknowledged the weight, let it go, and chosen peace. But this is not the end—it's your entry point into a new dimension of living.

Now is the time to integrate, stabilize, and align.

🌱 HOW TO BREAK THE FAST (Spiritually & Physically)

Spiritual Transition:

- Sit in silence before breaking your fast. Reflect. Don't rush back into noise.
- Speak a personal declaration of completion and continuation, like:
- "I honor the work I have done. I carry this clarity with me. I am reborn and aligned."

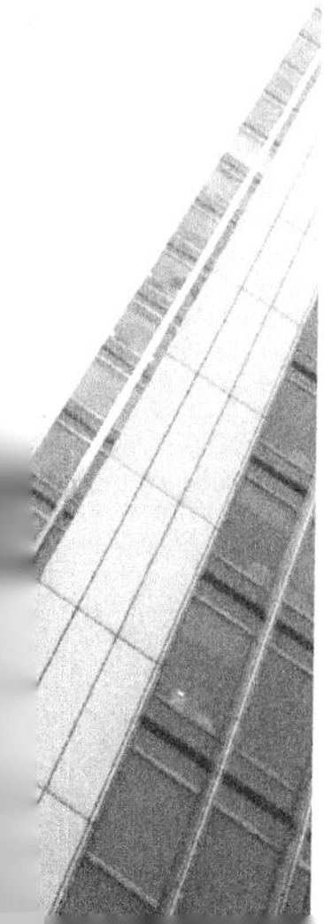

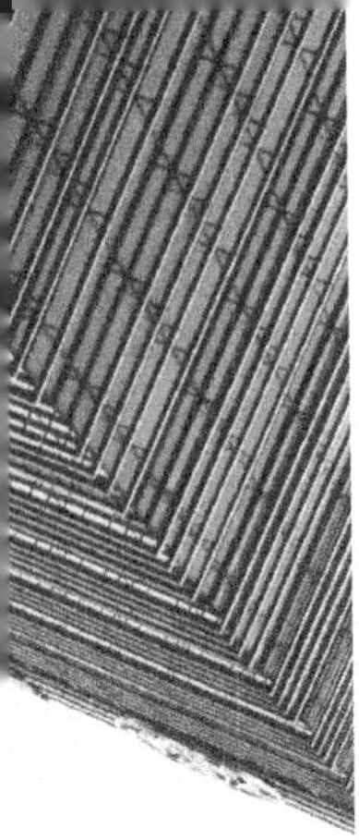

AFTER THE FAST:

- Light a candle, burn sage or incense, or use anointing oil to seal the new you.
- Write down what you are walking into. Set your next intention from a place of peace, not pressure.

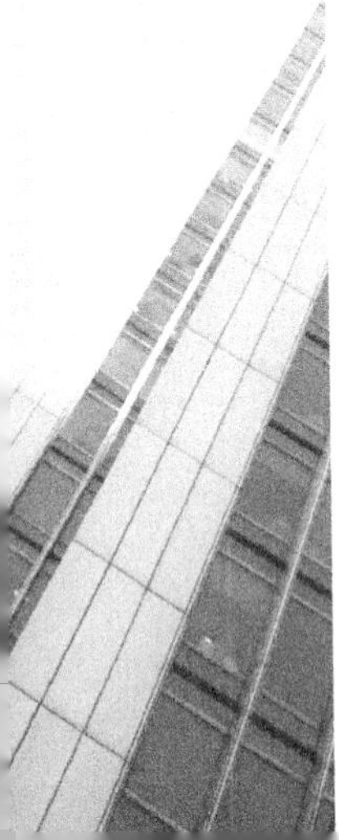

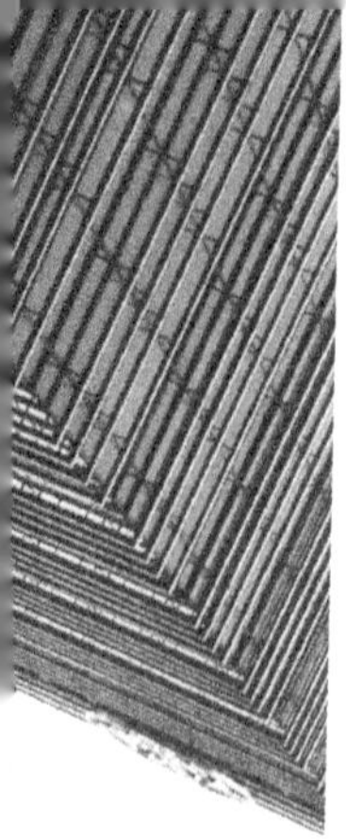

AFTER THE FAST:

AFTER THE FAST: Moving Forward in Power

Physical Reintroduction:

- Start light: fruit, warm herbal tea, soup, or smoothies to gently reawaken your body.
- Avoid heavy, fried, acidic, or over-processed foods for the first 12–24 hours.
- Drink alkaline or coconut water to rehydrate and restore your body's natural flow.

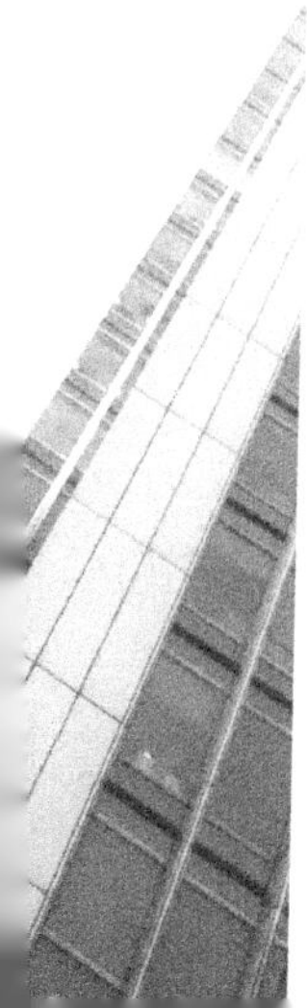

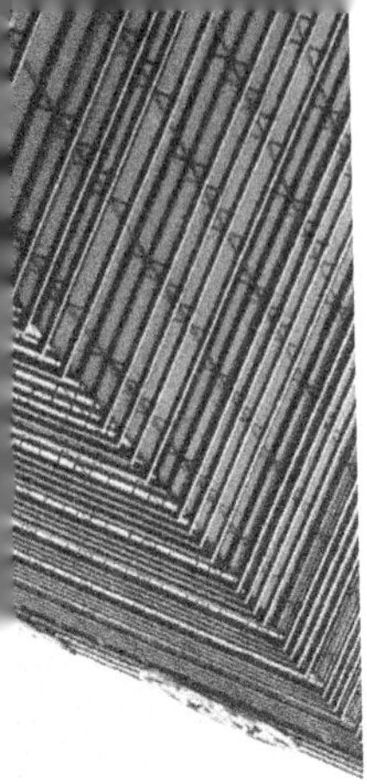

AFTER THE FAST:

WHEN TO REPEAT THIS FAST

This is a spiritual technology—sacred, effective, and personal. Repeat this 3-day fast:

- When you're manifesting something bold: a home, a vehicle, a major breakthrough.
- When facing impossibility: moments when it feels like "this is too big"—do it.
- When under spiritual or energetic attack: this fast centers and protects.
- When you're emotionally or spiritually exhausted: clarity returns here.
- Before making life-altering decisions: like marriage, separation, divorce, relocation.
- When you've outgrown someone you love: and must make a tough choice.

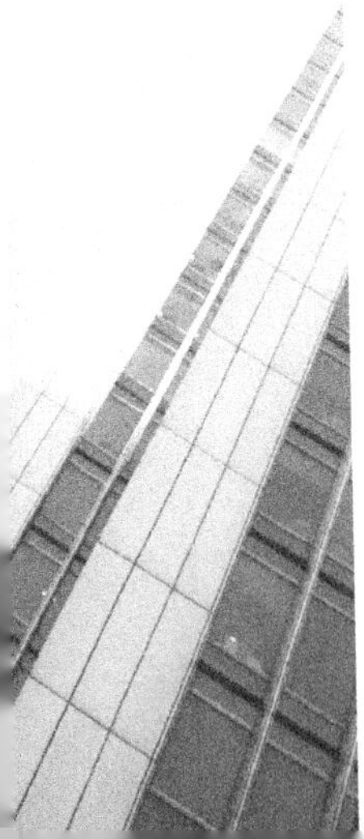

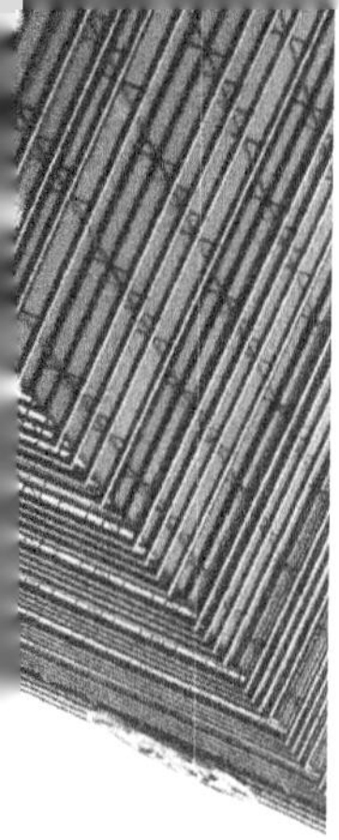

AFTER THE FAST:

- When you're letting go of people you deeply care for: and need divine strength.
- When peace seems far: this fast realigns your spirit with peace as your home.
- Whenever you're disconnected from self or Source: this is your reset button.

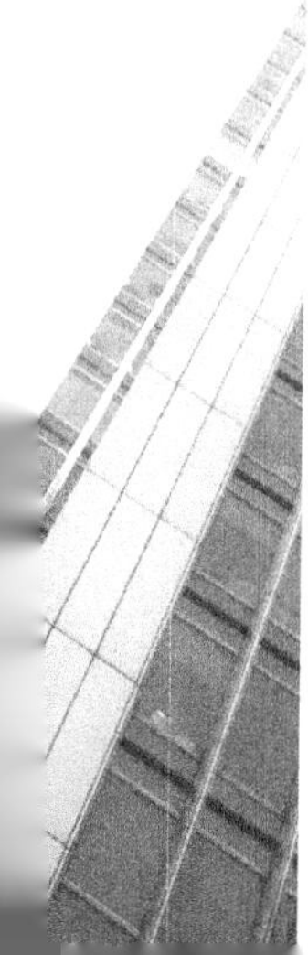

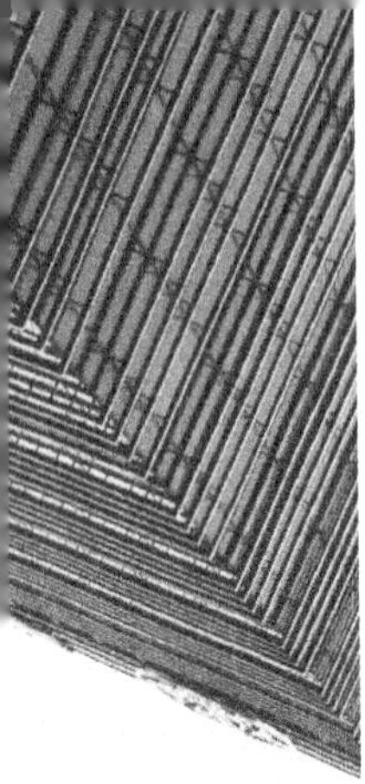

AFTER THE FAST:

NAVIGATION TO STAY ALIGNED

1. Stop chasing people's approval.

- Not everyone will understand your shift.
- You are not here to be palatable—you are here to be powerful.

2. Listen to you.

- Make space to learn from your own patterns.
- The divine speaks through your lived experience.

3. Recognize when you're people-pleasing.

- People-pleasing is self-abandonment in disguise.
- If pleasing them costs your peace, it's not worth the price.

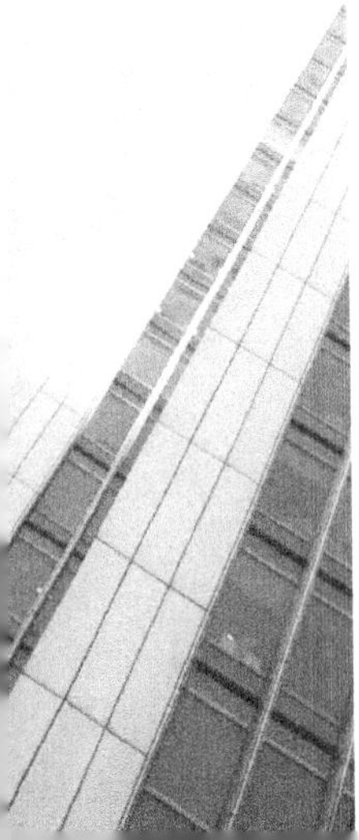

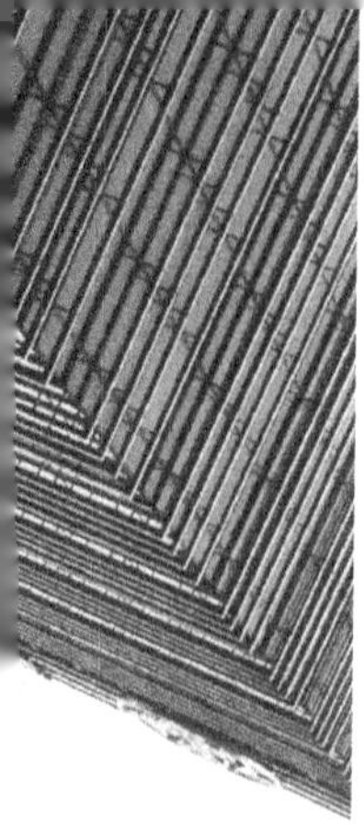

AFTER THE FAST:

4. Celebrate your peace.

- Peace is not the absence of problems—it is the presence of power.
- When peace becomes your normal, chaos will feel foreign.

5. Vibrate Higher and Stay There.

- Raise your frequency through:
    - Gratitude
    - Discipline
    - Nature
    - Prayer
    - Boundaries
    - Silence
    - Nourishment
    - Stillness
    - Truth-telling
    - Self-celebration

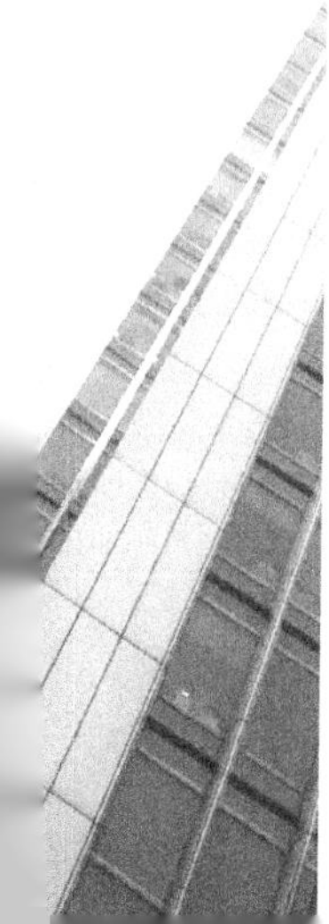

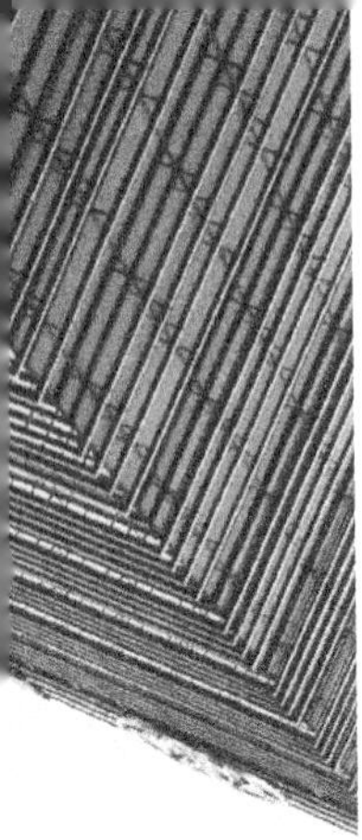

AFTER THE FAST:

Final Reflections

Many people try to "go with the flow" but they aren't even present.

They are empty vessels, reacting instead of living.

But you—you are awake now.

You are not lost.
You are not broken.
You are not too late.

You are a living altar.

A sacred flame.
A walking miracle.

This fast was not about performance. It was about presence.

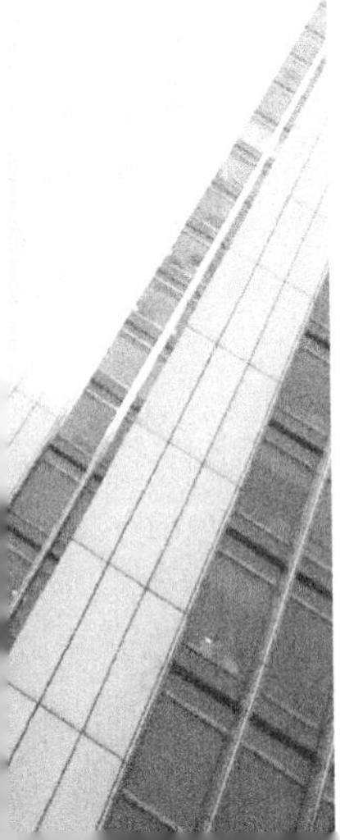

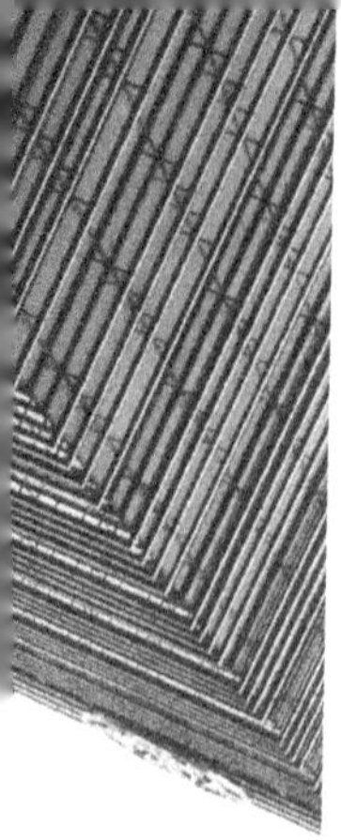

AFTER THE FAST:

FINAL DECLARATIONS

"I move forward not in fear, but in knowing."

"I am aligned with peace, and I protect my peace."

"I no longer beg for belonging—I belong to myself."

"I do not chase—I attract, I receive, I walk in readiness."

"My peace is not accidental. It is chosen, claimed, and celebrated."

"I vibrate higher, and I stay there. Not because it's easy, but because I'm worth it."

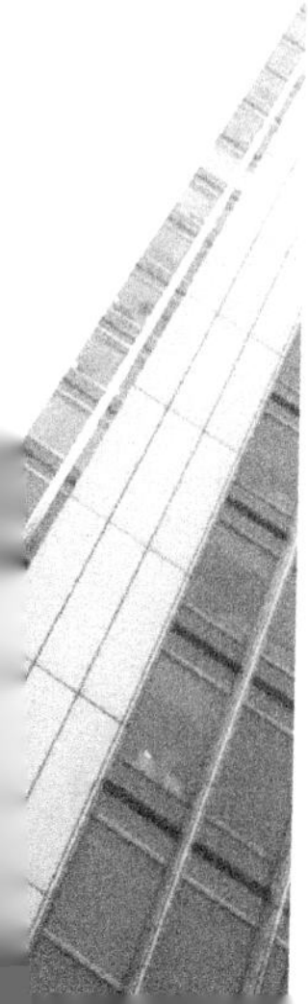

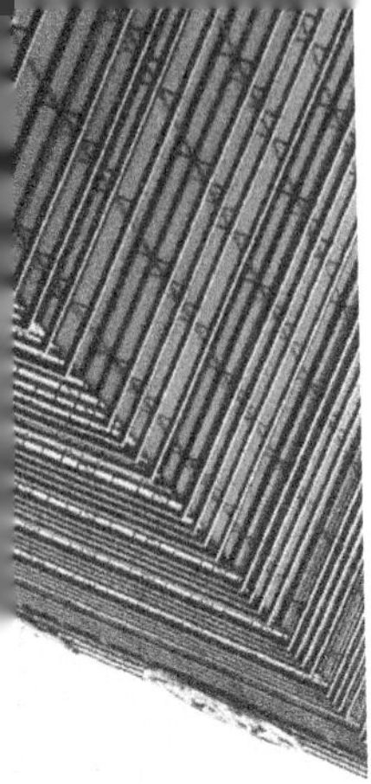

AFTER THE FAST:

To move on from now on, after completing this 3-day fast, you must adopt a sacred, sovereign, and steady attitude—one that reflects the transformation you've just undergone.

This is not just a mindset—it's a posture, a new way of being.

Attitude to Move Forward With

1. Gratitude as Your Ground

Attitude: "Nothing is owed to me, and yet everything is available to me."

- Be thankful not just for the good but for what grew you.
- Start each day saying: "Thank you for what was, thank you for what is, and thank you for what's becoming."

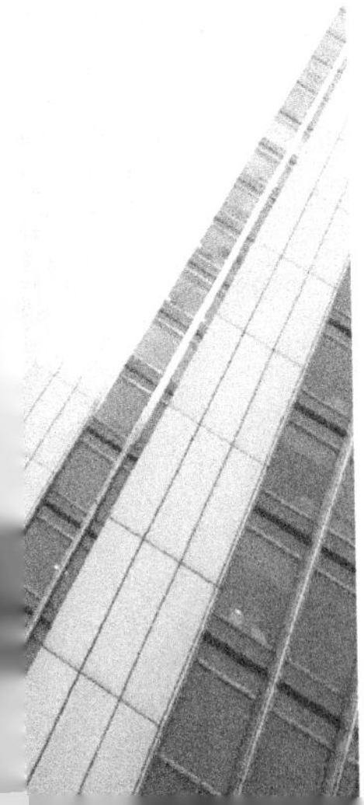

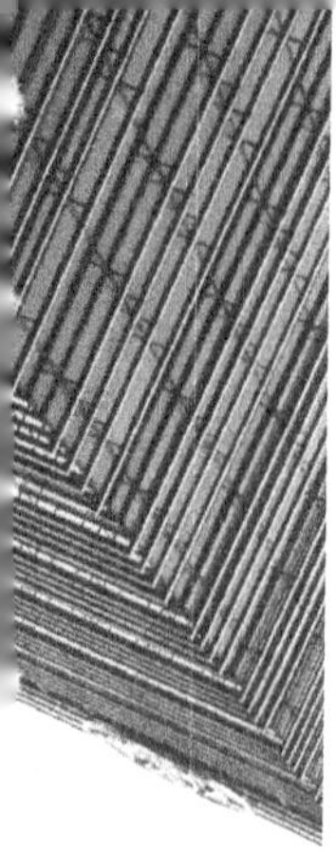

AFTER THE FAST:

2. Certainty Over Seeking

Attitude: "I am no longer hoping—I am walking in the knowing."

- Stop asking if you're ready—you are.
- You don't need outside confirmation. Trust what the fast revealed.
- Your healing is not a question, it's a declaration.

3. Peace as Priority

Attitude: "If it costs me my peace, it is too expensive."

- Don't negotiate your peace for people, places, or possibilities.
- Learn to walk away before you're broken.
- Choose stillness over chaos, alignment over attention.

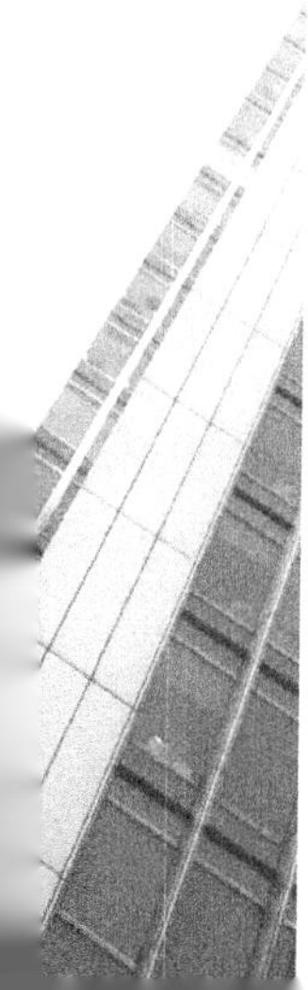

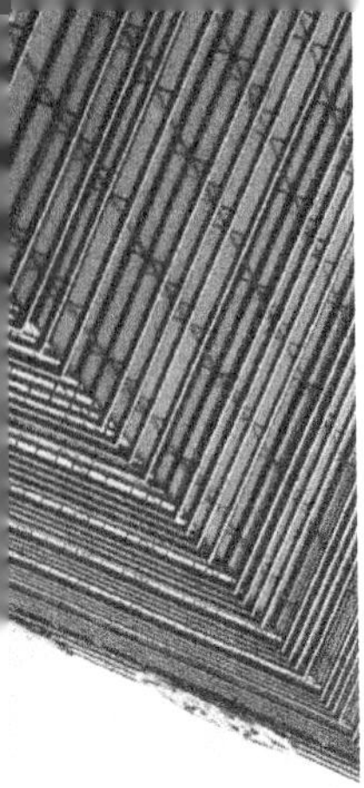

AFTER THE FAST:

4. Sovereignty and Self-Belonging

Attitude: "I belong to myself before I belong to anyone else."

- People-pleasing is over. Let them misunderstand you.
- You are not meant to fit—you're meant to lead.
- Sit with yourself. Choose yourself. Trust yourself.

5. Flow With Discernment

Attitude: "I flow, but I do not float aimlessly."

- Flow doesn't mean follow—it means align.
- Be soft but never spineless. Be open but not porous.
- You now know the difference between surrender and self-sabotage.

6. Boldness in Boundaries

Attitude: "My boundaries are not walls—they are bridges to freedom."

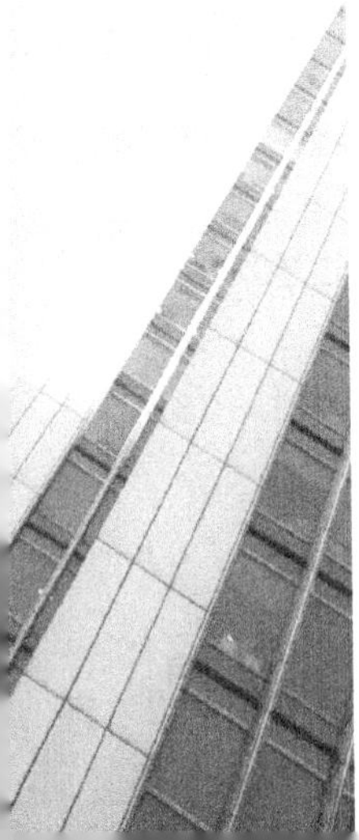

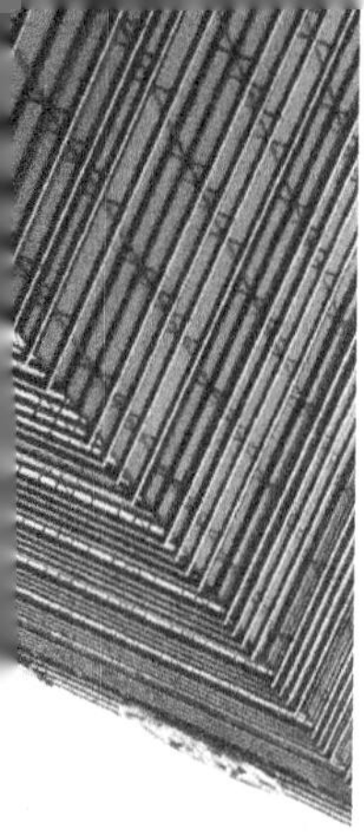

AFTER THE FAST:

- Let "no" be sacred.
- You don't owe access to anyone just because you love them.
- Boundaries protect the miracle you've just birthed.

7. Celebration Without Permission

Attitude: "I will no longer wait for applause—I celebrate myself."

- Clap for yourself before the world sees your worth.
- Take up space without apology. Be too much. Be full.
- Joy is your birthright—don't postpone it waiting for validation.

8. Divine Alignment Over Distraction

Attitude: "I live aligned with my divine design, not public opinion."

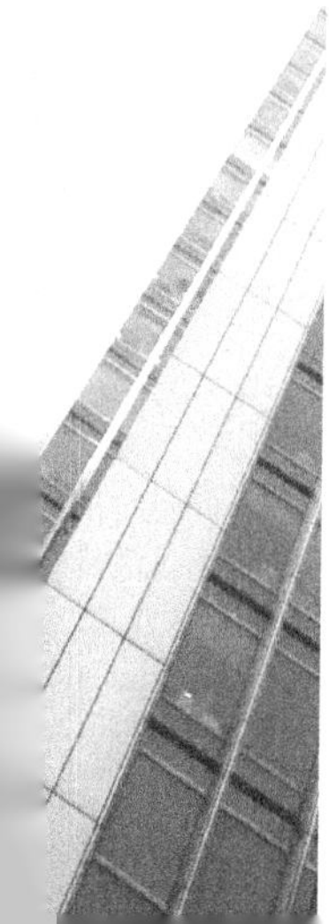

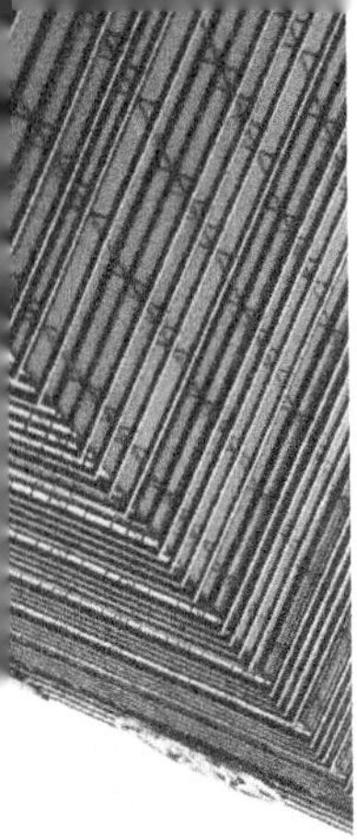

AFTER THE FAST:

- Stay close to Source. Don't let noise override the inner whisper.
- Let intuition lead your actions. Let spirit guard your decisions.
- You are not doing life alone—you're co-creating with divinity.

One Declaration to Carry Daily:

"I am at peace. I am in alignment. I am becoming more of who I was always meant to be."

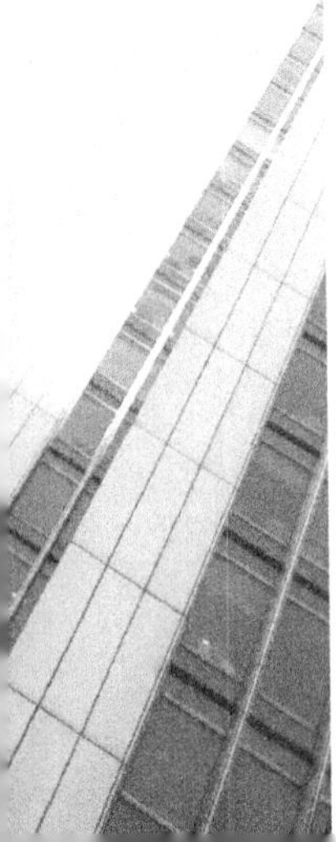

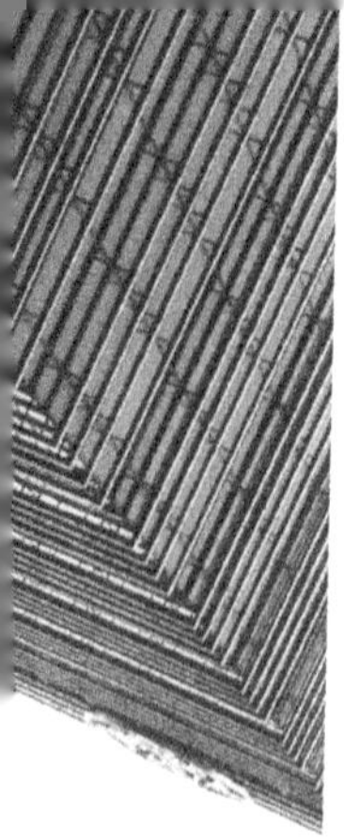

FINAL REMINDERS AND POWERFUL REINFORCEMENTS TO COMPLETE THIS JOURNEY AND ANCHOR YOUR TRANSFORMATION:

AFTER THE FAST: LIVE THE FAST

This wasn't just a 3-day event—it's a way of life now.

You didn't just stop eating.
You stopped feeding the things that were feeding off you.

Now:

- Don't go back to what you fasted from emotionally or spiritually.
- Don't reattach to what you cut cords from.
- Don't apologize for the clarity you gained.

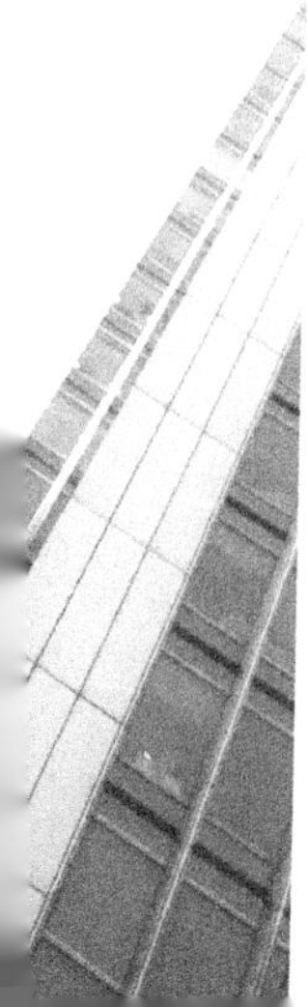

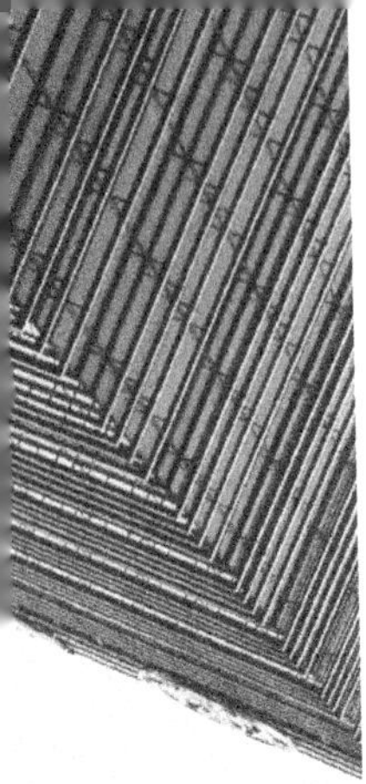

YOU ARE A NEW CODE

YOU ARE A NEW CODE

Your energy, mindset, and vibration have shifted.

So:

- New boundaries are necessary.
- New behaviors are required.
- New environments will support you best.

Let people meet the new you at the new level.

Not everyone can come. And that's okay.

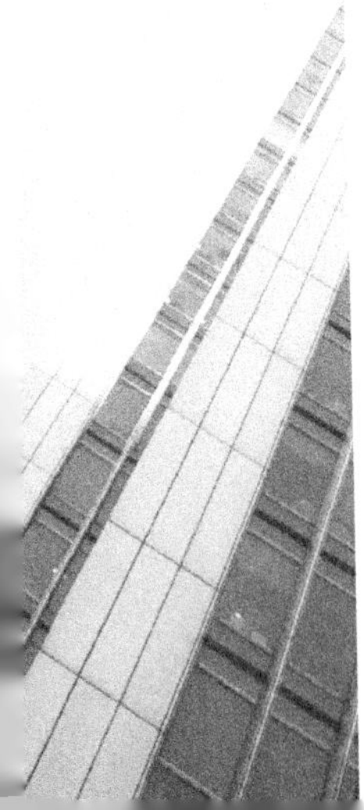

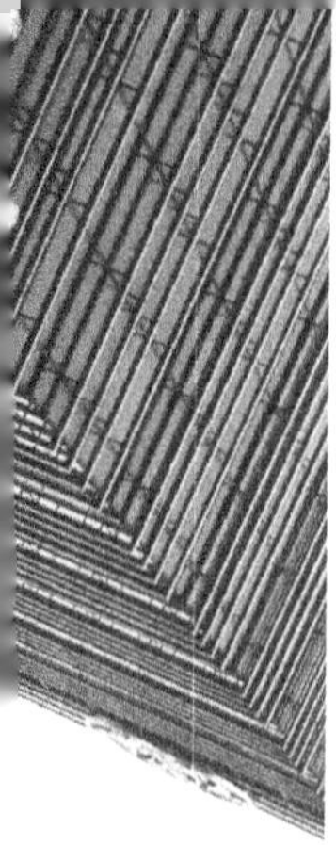

WHEN TO REPEAT THE 3-DAY FAST

WHEN TO REPEAT THE 3-DAY FAST

Do it again when:

- You're at a spiritual crossroads (career, relationship, identity shift).
- You feel heavy, stuck, confused, or under spiritual/psychic attack.
- You're initiating a big manifestation (new home, car, creative project, divine partnership).
- You need clarity about a major life decision (e.g. divorce, relocation, separation).
- You're grieving a version of yourself or others that you've outgrown.

Let it be your reset, your realignment, your recommitment.

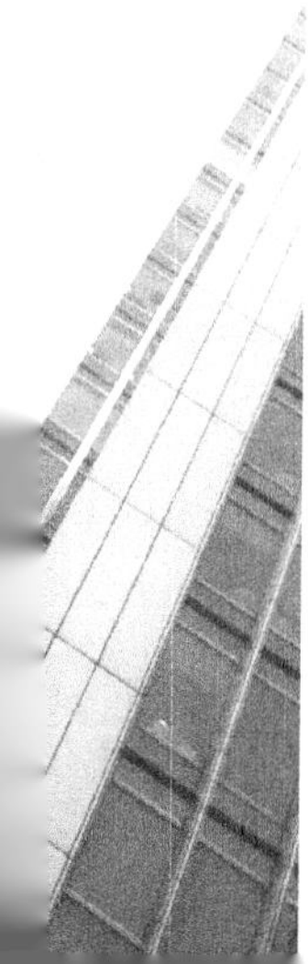

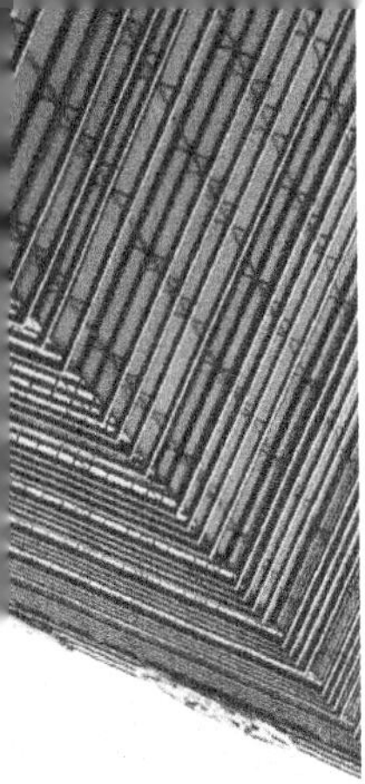

WARNING: DO NOT CHASE

WARNING: DO NOT CHASE

- Stop chasing closure, attention, validation, or explanations.
- Anyone who needs you to shrink, suppress, or suffer is not for you.
- You are no longer begging to belong. You already do.

STAYING IN HIGH VIBRATION

- Pray or meditate each morning—even if for 5 minutes.
- Keep affirming: "Peace is my baseline, not my reward."
- Keep your body light, your heart open, your space clean.
- Take spiritual baths, journal weekly, check in with your higher self often.
- Keep speaking to yourself with reverence and respect.

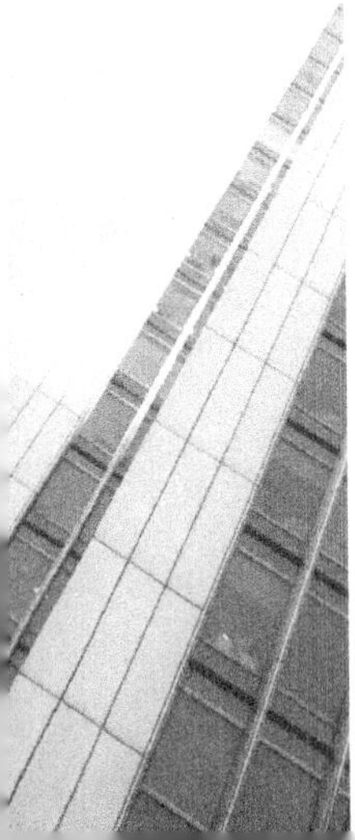

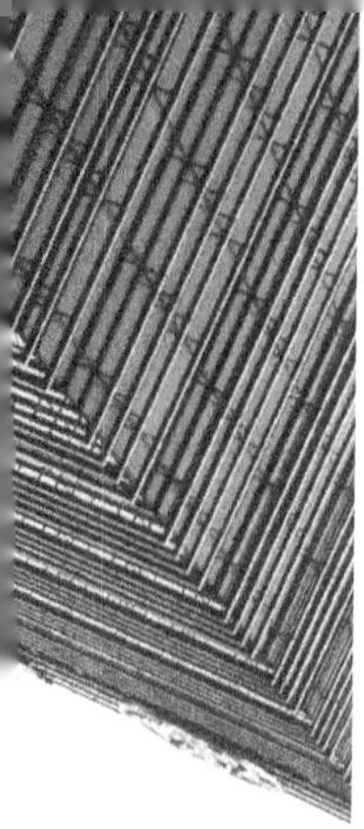

FINAL DECLARATION

FINAL DECLARATION

"From this day forward, I will not shrink to soothe others. I walk in full divine truth, aligned, protected, and unapologetically whole. My past is honored. My future is welcomed. My present is sacred."

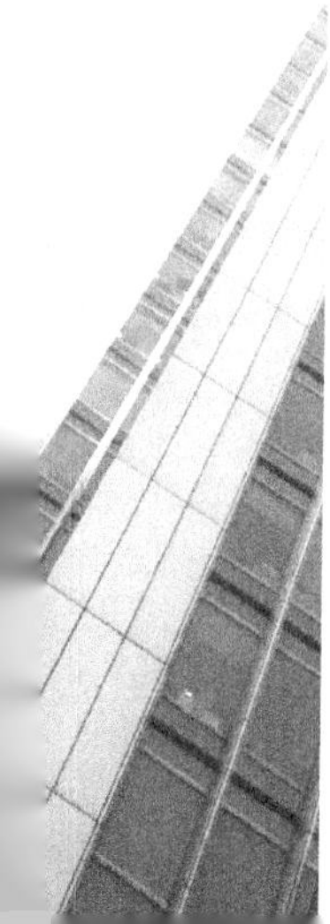

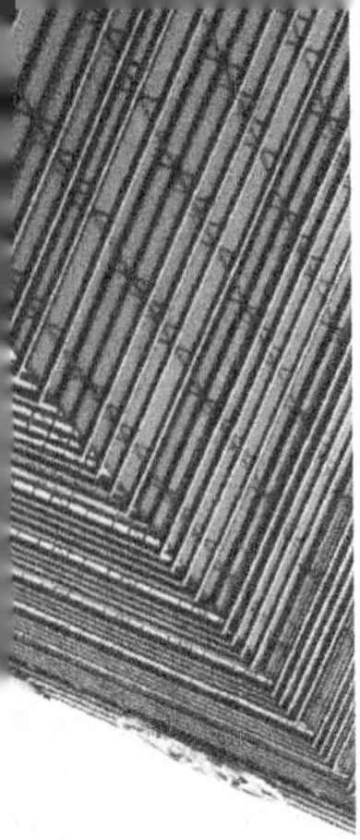

CLOSING RITUAL:

CLOSING RITUAL: "Breaking the Fast, Sealing the Shift"

This ritual is simple, sacred, and powerful.

It honors your body, soul, and spirit as you exit the fast.

Supplies Needed:

- 1 white candle (purity & clarity)
- 1 gold or yellow candle (divine power & joy)
- A bowl of clean water (symbol of spirit & rebirth)
- Your gratitude-based meal (see below)
- A journal or sacred paper
- Matches/lighter
- Optional: A soft instrumental playlist, essential oils (like frankincense, rose, or lavender)

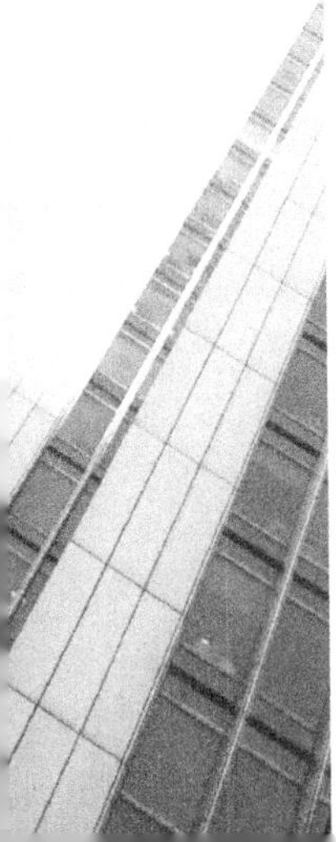

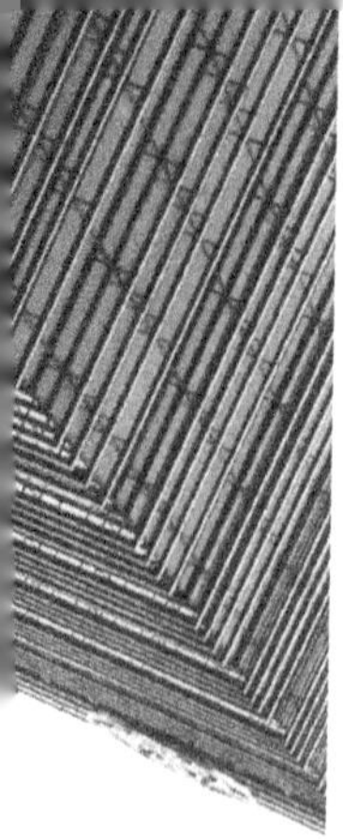

CLOSING RITUAL:

STEP 1: Light the Candles

Say aloud:

"I light this flame to symbolize my return—
not to who I was, but to who I truly am.

I call in clarity, joy, protection, and divine alignment.

I give thanks for the cleansing of my soul,
the healing of my heart,
and the rising of my spirit.

Let what was broken be sealed,
what was lost be found,
and what was denied be now declared."

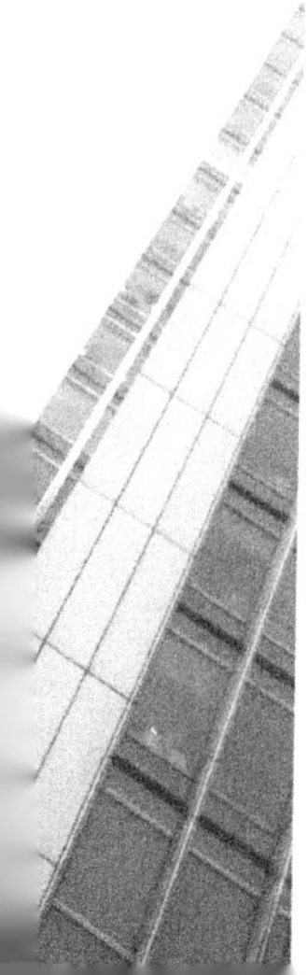

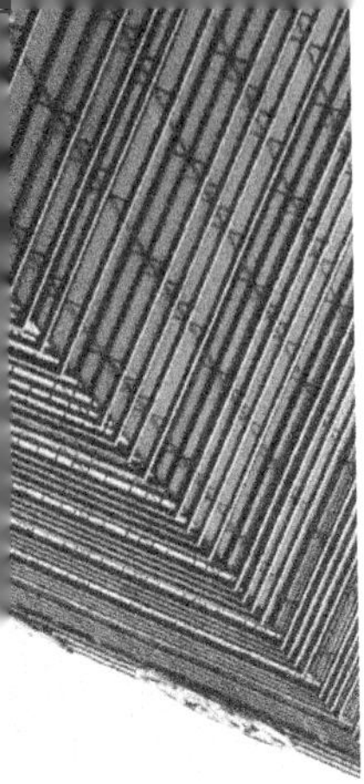

CLOSING RITUAL:

STEP 2: Water Activation

Dip your fingers into the bowl of water.

Rub it over your heart, crown, and wrists.

Say:

I anoint myself with this living water—
may I remain fluid, free, and full of peace.

Adjye! Asé. Amen. So it is."

Let the bowl sit beside you throughout your meal or journal time.

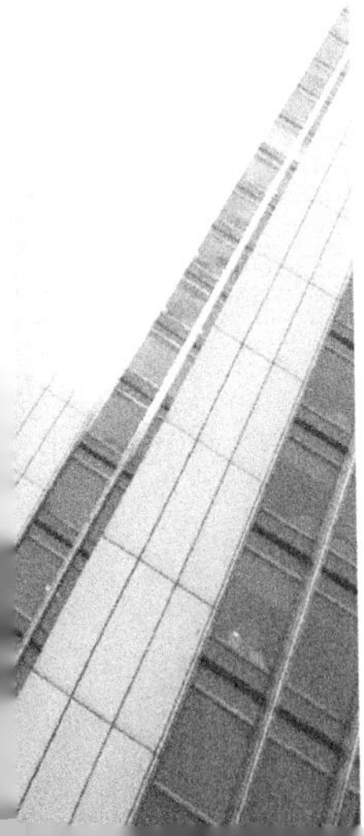

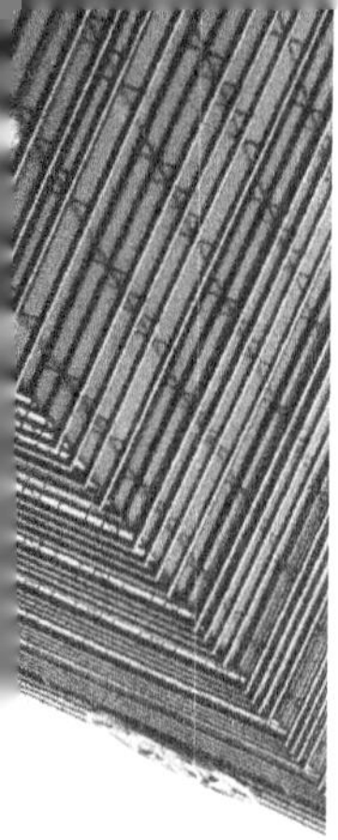

CLOSING RITUAL:

STEP 3: Read Your Declaration (aloud)

Write or read a final declaration. Here's a sample:

"I am no longer who I was.
I do not return to former patterns.

I vibrate at a new level of love,
peace, and divine power.

My soul is healed.
My vision is clear.

I am whole.
And I walk forward in trust."

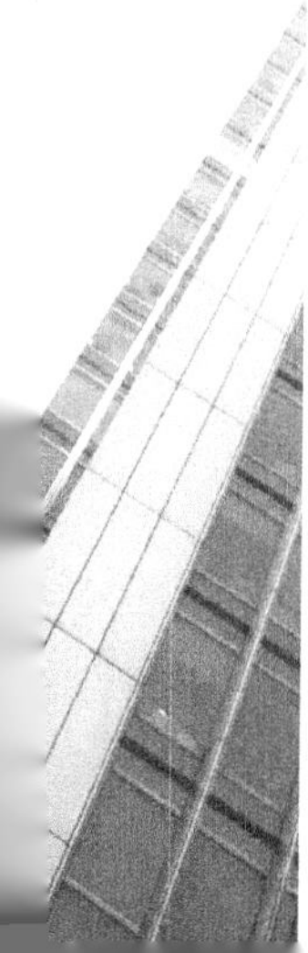

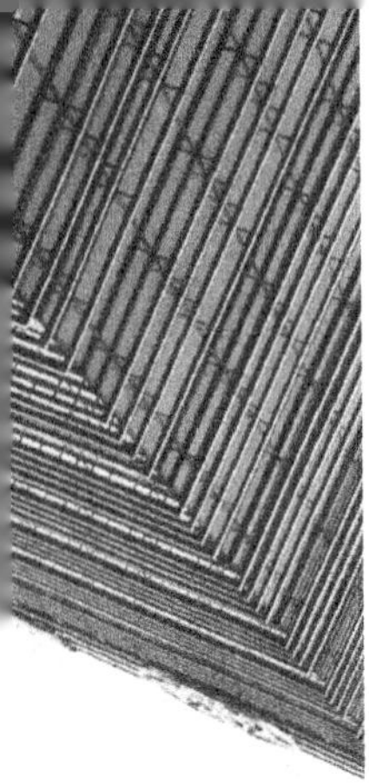

GRATITUDE-BASED MEAL PRAYER

Prepare a light, nourishing meal (fruit bowl, greens, whole grains, soup, or alkaline meal).

Before eating, place your hands over your food and say:

"I bless this meal with gratitude.

It is more than nourishment; it is a celebration of rebirth.

As this food enters my body, I honor every cell that held me through this fast.

I give thanks for my spirit, for the strength I did not know I had.

I eat with awareness.

I chew with reverence.

I digest with joy.

Let this meal remind me: I am alive, and I am aligned.

Asé. Amen. So it is."

Eat slowly. Breathe. Savor. Let this be ceremonial.

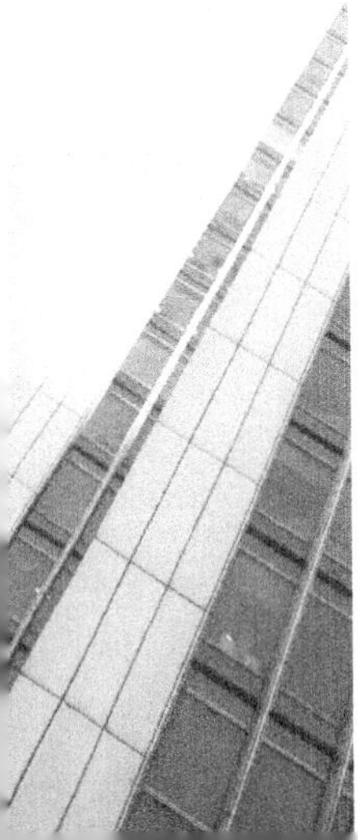

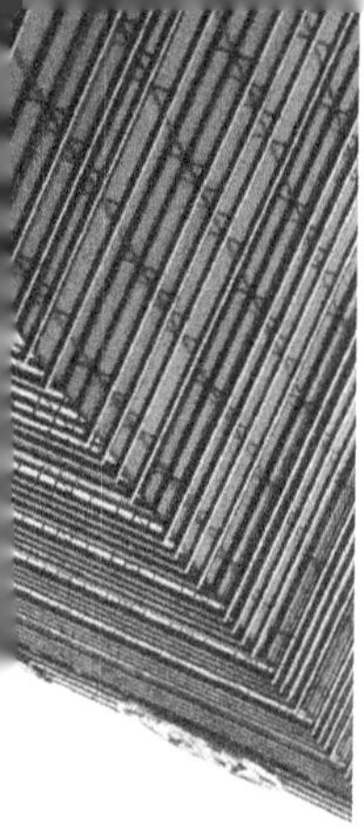

FINAL CANDLE MOMENT:

FINAL CANDLE MOMENT: “Closing the Circle”

Once you finish eating or journaling, gaze into the flame and say:

“The light I see before me is the light within me.
May it never dim. May it never break.
I am not returning—I am rising.
And I carry this flame with me into all things.
The fast is over, but the frequency remains.
I am whole. I am home.”

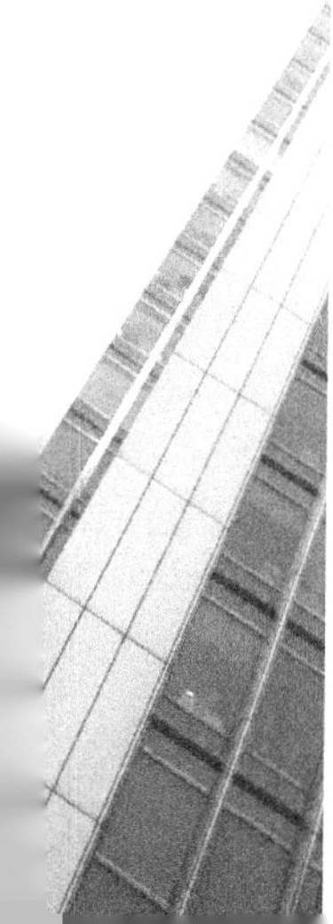

Put out the candle gently, or let it burn safely until it extinguishes on its own.
It is best to pinch the candlelight out instead of blowing them out which is considered as blowing away part of your essence or soul.

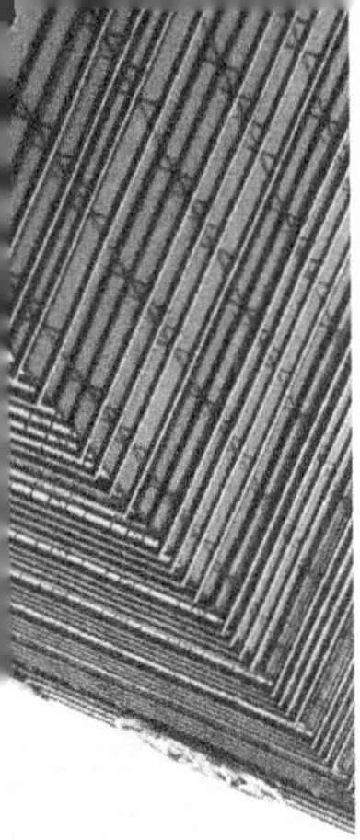

FINAL WORDS: CONCLUSION

Final Words: Conclusion of the Fast

You have not just completed a fast—
You have completed a spiritual shift.

You answered the call to pause, to purge, to listen deeply, and now you walk forward lighter, wiser, and more awake.

This was never about skipping food.
This was about feeding the soul.
This was never about deprivation.
It was about transformation.

You stood still so that your spirit could catch up.

You went within so that your truth could speak louder than your fears.
You fasted not to escape the world, but to remember you were never of it.

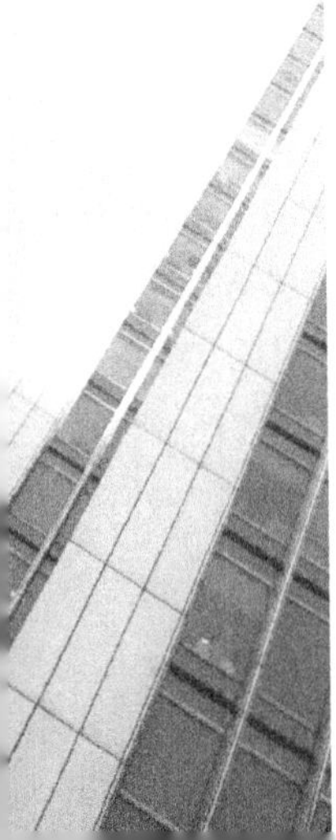

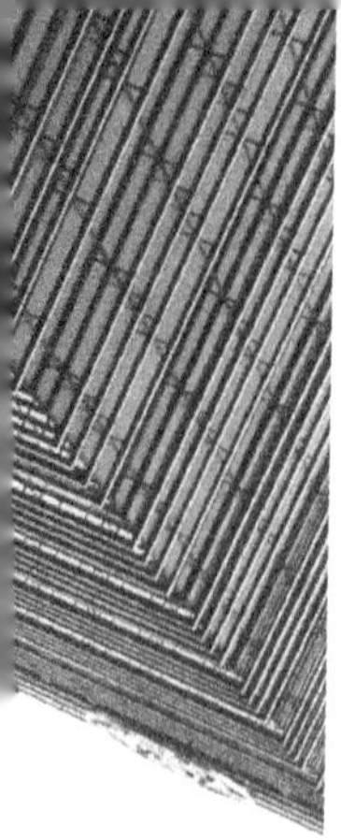

FINAL WORDS: CONCLUSION

You have confronted the past, sealed the unnecessary, and called forth the sacred future.

You have walked through the valley and emerged with clarity, not confusion—
with peace, not pain—
with purpose, not people-pleasing.

From this moment forward:

- Walk like your prayers are already answered.
- Speak like your words are spells (because they are).
- Breathe like you are aligned with the Divine.
- Move like peace is your default and joy is your companion.

Remember this:

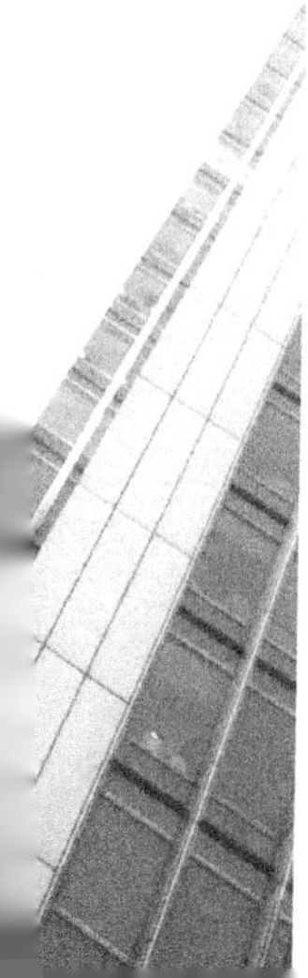

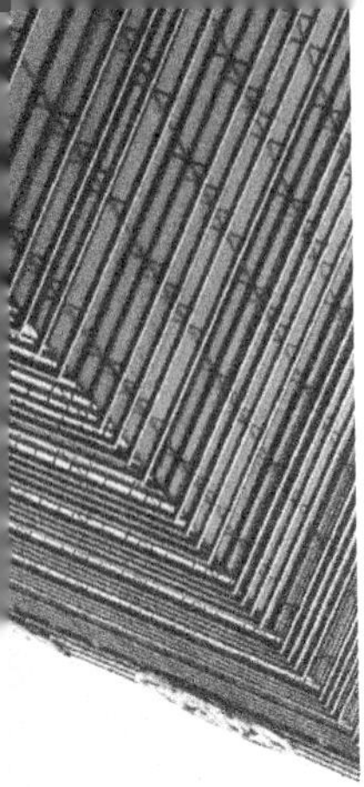

FINAL WORDS: CONCLUSION

Remember this:

- You do not need anyone's permission to be whole.
- You do not need their validation to exist.
- You are no longer available for chasing or convincing.
- You are no longer begging to be seen. You see yourself now.
- What you feel, sense, and know is real. Trust it.

Let peace be your proof.
Let alignment be your strategy.
Let divine timing be your rhythm.
Let love be your first and final answer.
This is your new beginning.
Live like it.
You are not who you were.
And that is the point.

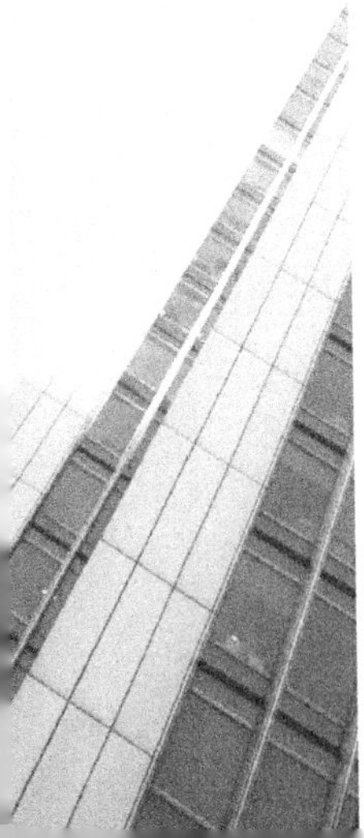

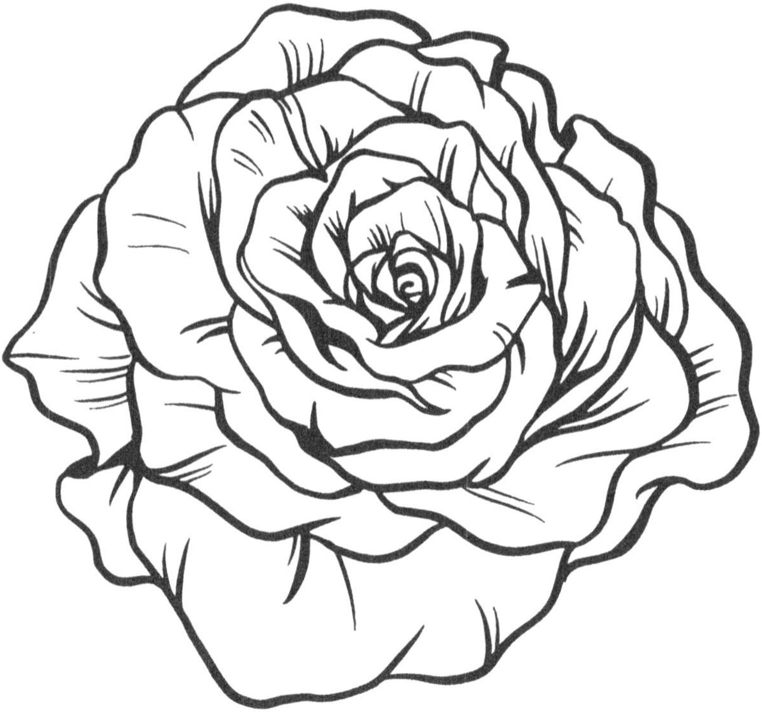

NOTES

NOTES

NOTES